SUPPORT WORKER TRAINING:

A GUIDE FOR HEALTH CARE PROFESSIONALS

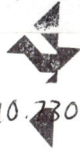

SUPPORT WORKER TRAINING:
A GUIDE FOR HEALTH CARE PROFESSIONALS

TERRY CHANDLER RMN, RGN, DipN, Cert Ed, RNT
Director of Staff Development and Training
Stockport, Tameside and Glossop College of Nursing
Tameside General Hospital,
Ashton-under-Lyne, UK

with contributions by:

John Dean RGN, Cert Ed, RNT
Head of Common Foundation Studies
York and Scarborough College of Midwifery and Nursing

Hilary Hampson RGN, Dip N (Part A), FETC, RCNT,
RNT, Cert Ed, IC Cert, SCM, B Ed
Development Officer for Quality
Tameside and Glossop Health Authority

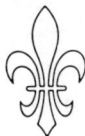

Baillière Tindall Limited

London   Philadelphia   Toronto   Sydney   Tokyo

Baillière Tindall
W.B. Saunders

24–28 Oval Road
London NW1 7DX

The Curtis Center
Independence Square West
Philadelphia, PA 19106–3399, USA

55 Horner Avenue
Toronto, Ontario, M8Z 4X6, Canada

Harcourt Brace Jovanovich Group
(Australia) Pty Ltd
30–52 Smidmore Street
Marrickville
NSW 2204, Australia

Harcourt Brace Jovanovich Japan Inc
Ichibancho Central Building,
22–1 Ichibancho
Chiyoda-ku, Tokyo 102, Japan

A catalogue record for this book is available from the British Library

ISBN 0–7020–1562–8

Typeset by Photo·graphics, Honiton, Devon
Printed in Great Britain by Clays Ltd, St Ives plc

Contents

Acknowledgements

In preparing this book many people contributed ideas and opinions which were gratefully accepted and used to form the basis of the text. I would like to express my thanks to them, including the staff of Tameside and Glossop Health Authority and the Joint Awarding Bodies for their literature which gave me many hours of reading. In particular I would like to express my sincere thanks to John Dean for writing Chapter 1 and Hilary Hampson for Chapter 7.

Finally I would like to thank Helena Hall for undertaking the daunting task of deciphering my writing, transposing it on to the word processor and where necessary, rearranging words and checking spelling.

Terry Chandler

Each year over 1 million vocational qualifications are awarded to people in a wide range of occupations. These qualifications are wide ranging and often confusing to both the employee and the employer, who discriminates in favour of personally known and often academic qualifications.

The purpose of this short book is to give the reader a little more insight into the whole issue surrounding the introduction of a new helper into health care.

Introduction

When preparing to put pen to paper to produce this book I was reminded of the Woody Allen film 'Everything you always wanted to know about sex but were afraid to ask'! I hasten to add that the content bears no relation to the title of the film. However, it did give me the idea that there are numerous questions related to the training of workers in support roles within health care that require an answer, or where no answer exists, at least some clarification. With this in mind I approached many friends and colleagues to find out what they know about training of support workers and the complexity of surrounding bodies involved in the evolution of this new role. Not surprisingly, we were in the same boat in that we knew a little bit about a lot of things but not a lot about individual areas. This book will unravel some of the mysteries surrounding Health Care Support Workers and hopefully will obviate the need for you to wade through the abundance of literature provided by the National Council for Vocational Qualifications (NCVQ) and the Joint Awarding Bodies and possibly drown in the sea of information. It is not intended as the definitive document but is intended to be a 'springboard' from which you can dive into the 'pool' of vocational qualifications from which you can emerge and after a brisk rub down with the towel of experience may spur you on to take a further dip and a longer swim! In essence you should be able to dip in and out of the book at will and hopefully be more able to guide those who want to learn to swim but are not sure what it entails, how to do it or how learning to swim can change their lives.

Some of the questions asked about the issues surrounding support roles give some indication of the direction of the book. One of the common questions asked is 'who are the Support Workers or Health Care Assistants, where will they come from and what will they do?' This question is dealt with later in the

Introduction and is reflective of the author's interpretation which may not necessarily align with views held by others. This area is one where many views are held and many reservations voiced as to the role and function of these workers in relation to the nursing and other health care professions as a whole. Some fall very positively on the side of the Introduction, some hold a very different and opposing view – others are in between with no firm conviction for or against the introduction but wait in limbo to either be convinced or say 'I told you so!'

The health care task force, having been alerted to the introduction of a 'New Helper Grade' (United Kingdom Central Council for Nursing, Midwifery and Health Visiting, 1986), has its own interpretation of the role and function, and in many instances can identify what the supportive role is that it would require from this worker. It all appeared relatively simple in the minds of many until other agencies with a vested interest in the taskforce of the UK, such as the National Health Service Training Authority, Care Sector Consortium, Central Council for Education and Training in Social Work, City and Guilds of London Institute, Business and Technical Education Council, entered the arena. This led to many questions being asked about how this massive jigsaw would piece together. Certain interested parties were advantaged in some respect in relation to the Joint Awarding Bodies involved, such as the Business and Technical Education Council, City and Guilds of London Institute, Central Council for Education and Training in Social Work, who will validate some of the course. Unless you were involved with or had experience of these, it seemed to be a complicated and complex system. Unfamiliar words and phrases appeared in our daily vocabulary such as National Vocational Qualification, Accreditation of Prior Learning, Employment Training and Enterprise Councils. These areas all became part of the issues related to the introduction of a 'new worker'.

The question of how they all fit together is still somewhat puzzling. Other interested parties also add to the confusion of the situation – who or what is the National Health Service Training Authority? The Care Sector Consortium? What do they do and how do they figure in this? Perhaps by 'dipping' into the relevant 'lanes' a little underwater light may be shed into what may seem very deep water to those somewhat reluctant to swim. The starter pistol is raised – on your marks!

With the publication by the UKCC in 1986 of the proposals for a reform of nursing in terms of practice and education – Project 2000 (see Chapter 2) – many questions were raised by the nursing profession regarding the recommendations, and not least by the recommendation that 'there should be a new helper directly supervised and monitored by the registered practitioner'. Various titles were given to this 'new' grade. In the document itself the title 'aide' is used. This was then altered to 'Support Worker' – which in reality is a description of the role they would adopt rather than a title. There are in existence numerous Support Workers such as Porters, Domestic Workers, Ward Clerks, Nursing Auxiliaries and many others. In the past new roles within the caring teams have arisen as a result of problems in recruiting and in some instances the roles have been imposed.

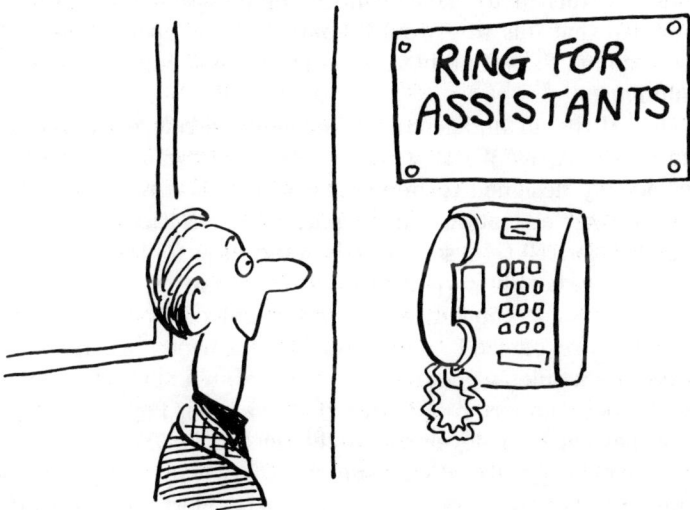

The situation today is different in that the profession has been consulted, and has indeed been encouraged, to be actively involved in the determination of this new helper role. Much has been written both for and against the formulation and introduction of a new grade of helper. Some see this role as a totally nursing orientated role and elements of 'nursing' hived off to give to them. Others see this as a great opportunity to provide the qualified practitioner with a trained helper who will contribute effectively to the team and will allow the qualified practitioner the time to undertake that at which he or she is expert, e.g. nursing. One could argue that by doing this we are allowing nursing to be short changed but the fact remains that the professionals are in a position to determine the exact nature of the role and function of this new worker and by doing so could prevent this occurrence. In an ideal situation all nursing activities would be undertaken by the qualified practitioners – in the harsh reality this is not necessarily the case. In certain areas much of the 'hands on' nursing activities are undertaken by untrained personnel with the qualified practitioner involved in the more technological aspects of the Nurse's role, supervising the activities of the taskforce. The concerns regarding this new role must not be underestimated and indeed many are valid, but the situation could be turned to the advantage of the profession. It is not intended that this role would replace or overlap the role of the professional Nurse but that it would provide a range of supporting functions.

One of the advantages of introducing the role is the fact that the Health Care Workers will undergo a training programme specifically designed to prepare them for their role. This is not professional education, but is part of the National Vocational Qualification (NVQ) system which would allow for freer movement within the health care sector. The system is based on the acquisition of competence and the award of credits towards a nationally recognized qualification (see Chapter 4). By adding different modules a person could move from a nursing-orientated role into a support role within, for example, Physiotherapy or they may wish to develop their clerical skills. The training for those working within these support roles will have a common core with add on 'units' or 'modules' particularly related to their chosen area of work.

Since the publication of Project 2000, the supportive roles have been a grey area. The role and function of this grade of Health Care Worker is crucial to the success of the new system of preparing the practitioners of the future. Since the initial discussions and proposals, much work has been undertaken to determine the competence levels required of the new grade. The

'Health Care Assistant' is now the name we have for the new grade, and is not a Nursing Auxiliary by another name. The Health Care Assistant will differ from the present Auxiliary in both the role and function within the care team. A major fundamental difference is that they will be specifically trained to undertake the job for which they are employed. The same principle applies to the Health Care Support Workers who in future will replace the unqualified workers in other health care settings, e.g. Physiotherapy, Social Services.

In a letter to the Health Authorities' General Managers the National Health Service Management Executive said, 'that by giving a more systematic training to support staff it may be possible to enhance the range of activities which may be safely delegated on the professional practitioner' and secondly 'by putting different competencies together in new ways, it may be possible to enhance the support which the non professional can offer.'

The specific role, job description, and the title by which the new worker will be known are to be determined at local level. What is required is flexibility, not only in relation to how the people who are to fill these roles will be prepared subsequently and developed, but also in relation to the role itself which of necessity must be adaptable to future trends and changes in the patterns of service delivery. There have been suggestions that the Health Care Assistant role should be generic, in that the person should be able to turn his or her hand to anything. However, this is impractical, although elements of commonality within the roles is inevitable. In developing the role of the Health Care Support Worker it is important to get it right, not only for the workers themselves but for the health care professions as a whole and more importantly the clients and patients for whom the service is provided.

1

Project 2000, A New Preparation for Practice

This opening chapter will provide an overview of one of the major factors in determining both the agenda and the timescale for the training of Health Care Support Workers. In doing so, it is recognized that the training of Health Care Support Workers is not only an issue for the nursing profession; it is of equal importance to the various other professions allied to medicine for whom an 'assistant' or 'helper' grade is considered necessary. It is not the intention to provide a comprehensive overview of Project 2000; that is beyond the scope of this book. This chapter serves to summarize those aspects of Project 2000 which are of most benefit to a discussion about the training of Health Care Support Workers.

In 1986, the United Kingdom Central Council for Nursing, Midwifery and Health Visiting (UKCC) published its report *Project 2000, A New Preparation for Practice*. At the time of publication it represented the result of 2 years of dedicated work, included the publication and widespread discussion of six project papers, and involved many different groups including the other statutory bodies for Nursing, Midwifery and Health Visiting, the nursing press and experts from outside the world of nursing. The scope for the consultation process was considerable. In her introductory message to the report, Audrey Emerton, the Chairman of the UKCC referred to this as:

> ... an exercise 'in the sunshine', and that the thinking underlying the Report and its preparation should be in the public arena as soon as possible to encourage discussion and debate. (UKCC, 1986)

The discussion and debate, sometimes very heated, has continued beyond the initial implementation of Project 2000. At the time of writing, each Health Region in the United Kingdom has at least one Nurse Education Centre delivering Project 2000 courses, in most regions there are already two, with approval in principle having been given to more. Still the arguments rage on about the respective merits of particular aspects of Project 2000.

Project 2000, arguably, represents the most wide ranging set of reforms in Nursing Education since the original 'Nurses Act' of 1919. It is not because of a lack of suggestions to reform the system that it has taken so long. Countless reports condemning one or more aspects of Nursing Education have been produced by a variety of different organizations and public bodies with, it could be argued, only cosmetic results. What makes these reforms different from previous attempts is that they were proposed by the elected representatives of the Nursing, Midwifery and Health Visiting professions. Unlike previous attempts at reform, this one has come from within rather than outside the professions.

The context within which Project 2000 was produced is very important in understanding the arguments for change. The case for change by this time was both convincing and complex.

> The case for change in the pattern of preparation for nursing, midwifery and health visiting at the present time is a many sided one. There is a case for change because of the educational difficulties of the present pattern. This has long been known, but it has been further highlighted and documented by the accumulating research evidence of the last ten years. There is a case for change because of the problems the present arrangements pose for service delivery, and in the likely increase in these problems in the light of present trends. There is also a case for change because present trends simply cannot continue. The supply of recruits is dwindling and will continue to do so. (UKCC, 1986, p. 9)

In presenting the case for change the point will be made that 'no change' was not an option at all. The 'no change' option had greeted many previous reports, notably the *Report of the Committee on Nursing (The Briggs Report)* in 1972 (HMSO, 1972). The problems that existed in Nursing Education continued to develop in the face of unprecedented change in the delivery of health care in the United Kingdom.

The Project 2000 report categorized the problems that existed in Nurse Education under a number of headings. It described the need for change in the context of 'A Changing World', 'Deficiencies from an Educational Viewpoint', 'Disadvantages from the Service

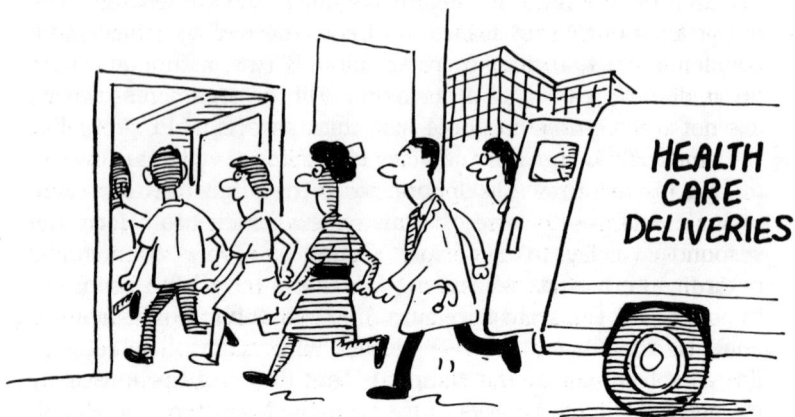

Standpoint', 'Problems of Recruitment' and 'Frustration Within The Profession'.

A changing world

Health care delivery takes place within a context, and that context is socially, culturally, economically and politically defined. Nurses are themselves part of society, the context, and it is with these considerations in mind that we need to view the changing world in which health care takes place.

The first thing that becomes apparent is that the need for health care is not likely to diminish. The types of health care demanded and the ability of the nation to respond to that demand might change, but the indications are that need will continue to increase. This represents a direct challenge to the assumption that underpinned the establishment of the National Health Service; that health care demands would diminish as a direct result of the establishment of this service.

Changing patterns of morbidity and mortality have been marked since 1948. In this time the impact of infective and parasitic diseases on the nation's health has declined considerably. The importance of these diseases has been replaced by other health problems which are largely preventable. These include coronary heart disease, cancer and accidents. The present arrangements are not well equipped to deal with these 'preventable' problems.

Demographic changes and class inequalities in terms of access to and provision of appropriate health care facilities represent major challenges to a health care system which has clearly not responded easily to the many reports and recommendations regarding both of these issues. *Inequalities in Health, The Black Report* (Townsend and Davidson, 1982) established that in some cases the 'health-gap' between classes has actually widened since the establishment of the National Health Service. Demographic changes are highlighting the increased need for respite care, and other forms of care for an elderly population which makes disproportionately high demands on health and social services.

An increasing awareness of how inappropriate wholesale institutional care is for many different client groups including the elderly, people with learning difficulties, the mentally ill and children, has resulted in a major review of health care facilities for these groups. In very general terms this has resulted in an increasing emphasis on care in the community setting, in the private and voluntary sectors and by informal carers at home.

In short, all health care professions need to be able to respond effectively to the health needs of a rapidly changing world, developing new skills when they are needed and abandoning obsolete practices when they are no longer required.

Deficiencies from an educational viewpoint

A Nurse Education system which is essentially based on a compromise between the educational needs of students and the constant pressure to provide Student Nurses as part of the workforce is fundamentally flawed (UKCC, 1986, p. 10).

Linked to the service need for a constant supply of new recruits to the profession is the 'constant grind' of many new student intakes per year, allowing teachers little time to reflect on their own practice and develop themselves and their resources as a result. The 'marriage' to the very real needs of the service has resulted in the educational needs of students being sacrificed on the altar of short-term health care provision, the demands of which are occasionally in direct conflict with the educational needs of the student.

National figures show a drop out rate of 15–20% with a further 15–20% failing to complete, successfully, their examinations, illustrating how poorly the Nurse Education system has served its students. Research into the individual experiences of some of those students reveals the extent to which the inadequate preparation, supervision and mentorship of students (Birch, 1975; Gott, 1984) has contributed to this disgraceful figure of 30–40% of Student Nurses failing to qualify.

Serious concern has also been expressed about the wasted opportunities for shared learning by Student Nurses studying different courses and the resources involved in running different courses which replicate each other for substantial periods of time. In addition to the wasted teaching resources that this entails, it further contributes to the isolationism, based on misunderstanding of other Nurses' roles, of the different specialisms within nursing.

Isolationism from other forms of 'post-school education' is an accusation which is made of pre-Project 2000 Nurse Education. Large numbers of school leavers have been undertaking their nursing qualifications isolated from other higher education and further education students. In addition to not mixing with other students, the nursing qualification itself has not been accorded any external educational value until very recently, outside the world of Nursing. Work by various organizations including the Open University, Sheffield City Polytechnic and the National Council for Vocational Qualifications (NCVQ) has begun to alter this situation so that pre-Project 2000 courses as well as Project 2000 courses may carry at least some credit towards other awards.

Disadvantages from the service standpoint

The use of Student Nurses as an integral part of the Nursing workforce has been an important and contentious aspect of their education since the establishment of modern Nurse Education in the early part of this century. As a compromise then it was understandable. As a continuing part of Nurse Education it makes little or no sense from a service point of view.

Continuity of care is difficult to establish in a ward or department when the largest part of the Nursing workforce is only there for between 4 and 12 weeks. At the end of the 'placement' in a clinical area the students are replaced by other students, all of whom will need to be orientated to this new environment. This system for staffing wards inevitably either takes up a lot of time of the 'permanent' staff which could otherwise be used for direct patient care, or it does not get done. Estimates vary as to how inefficient this system is. The Department of Health Project 2000 Implementation Group has estimated that replacing Student Nurses with more permanent staff should be up to 20% more efficient in manpower terms. In other words five whole time equivalent staff can be replaced in clinical areas by four whole time equivalent permanent staff. This is a rather crude simplification of a very complex issue and does not give due recognition to the wider issue of skill-mix but it serves to illustrate the inefficiency of staffing wards with short-term transient members of staff (Project 2000 Implementation Group, 1989).

Problems of recruitment

Problems of recruitment will remain if nursing continues to recruit mainly from the 18-year-old female school leaver cohort, and continues to lose valuable members of the profession by being unable to respond appropriately to their personal and professional needs.

Referred to variously as the 'demographic time-bomb' and the 'demographic black-hole', we have known for some considerable time that these prospective recruits have been diminishing in number since 1981 and are due to reach their lowest level in 1991. Suggested solutions to this problem include making Nursing Education accessible to mature entrants by, for example developing flexible courses which take into account the domestic commitments of potential students. Very closely linked to this is the need for a much more creative approach to employment arrangements so that highly educated and valuable staff are not lost to the National Health Service forever. Other groups of people who are under-represented and therefore represent a large pool of potential recruits to nursing include people from ethnic minority groups, married women and men.

We have already identified the problems facing family carers, usually daughters, in the event of an ageing population (Office of Population Censuses and Surveys, 1985). This means that at a time when we are trying to recruit older people into nursing, they themselves are increasingly likely to be involved in providing care for another family member. The need to make provision for members of staff for the care of older relatives as well as children will become increasingly important.

Frustration within the profession

For all of these and other reasons there is a great deal of anxiety about the preparation of Nurses, and the ability of the profession to respond to changing health needs. The Project 2000 group heard from many individuals and groups about the weaknesses and deficiencies in Nurse Education:

> People would speak of the weaknesses of initial nurse preparations as 'using students as pairs of hands'; they would criticise 'the gap between theory and practice'; they would refer to 'fragmentation' and 'divisions', 'overlap' between different programmes and the lack of a sense of progression in the many options on offer. (UKCC, 1986, p. 12)

Proposed solutions

Whilst the original Project 2000 recommendations have undergone a degree, (some people would say a considerable one), of modification since their initial publication in 1986, for the purposes of this book the essential recommendations have retained their significance in the implementation of Project 2000. This is not to deny that the 'interpretation' and 'translation' of those recommendations into reality have not been hotly debated and at times fiercely attacked and defended. On the contrary, some of the published major recommendations were subsequently rejected outright.

The first and most significant recommendation is that a new Registered Practitioner should be created whose vocational education prepares him or her to work in both institutional and non-institutional settings. In making this its first major recommendation the Project Group was clearly identifying that in order to respond appropriately to the changing health needs of people in the UK, the skills required by Nurses to work in newly defined areas would need to be reviewed. In many instances new areas of competence would need to be developed. These revised 'competencies' are now established, and are set out as training outcomes in the 'Training Rules' (HMSO, 1989).

If the 'product' of the education system is to change in a radical way, then the education 'process' cannot remain the same. Conversely if the Nurse Education system remains unaltered then the qualifying Nurse will be no more appropriately prepared than those we are educating at present.

One of the recurrent themes in the discussions leading up to the publication of Project 2000 and its subsequent implementation is that of the 'status of Student Nurses'. There are a number of different aspects to this particular issue, and it is around this issue that the discussions surrounding the nursing Health Care Support Worker begin to emerge.

In tackling the complex issue of the long-term educational needs of students versus the immediate needs of service in the delivery of care, the Project Group recommended that, for the full 3 years of the educational programme, Student Nurses should be 'supernumerary' to staffing establishments. This means that instead of wards and departments being dependent on Student Nurses for staffing them, the staffing establishment should be independent of them. This represents one of the key compromises between the original proposals and the implementation of Project 2000. Three years of supernumerary status has now been qualified by the words 'rostered contribution' and 'non-rostered' time. For 32 weeks, usually within the last year of the course, students will be required to make a 'rostered contribution' to the work of the ward or department. This time will continue to be education-ally led, the student must be supervised, but the student will be considered as part of the resources available for patient care delivery.

If Student Nurses are to be taken out of the workforce equation for a substantial part of their education, the significant contribution that they made in the past must be picked up by other staff. To this end the Project Group recommended that:

> There should be a new helper, directly supervised and monitored by a registered practitioner (UKCC, 1986, p. 70)

In making this recommendation the Project Group recognized the potential dilemma of making proposals about a grade of staff over which they would have no responsibility. They did state however that:

> ... it was incumbent upon us to be clear about the practitioner role, and to state the kind of help which was needed by the new practitioner, if a practitioner-centred division of labour were to become a working reality. (UKCC, 1986, p. 64)

They also recommended that the helper grade to which they referred should be trained, but that the training should be 'limited' and of direct relevance to the particular care setting that the helper is working in. Beyond this, the suggestions made about this particular grade of staff are, perhaps necessarily, vague. This vagueness extends even to the title. In *Project 2000, A New Preparation for Practice* they are referred to, variously, as 'helpers' and 'aides'. One of the recommendations that was made about the training of these 'aides' was that it should follow guidelines issued by the four National Boards for Nursing, Midwifery and Health Visiting. Events have subsequently over-taken this recommendation and these form the basis for other sections in this book. Recent communication, particularly from the National Health Management Executive, *Nurse Education and Training: Implementation of Project 2000 in 1990–91* has attempted to clarify the definition of the Health Care Assistant grades of staff and as such are much more illuminating than the original Project 2000 publication (Project 2000 Implementation Group, 1989).

The last area of the original recommendations that I would like to make specific reference to is that of the cessation of Enrolled Nurse training. Whilst this recommendation does not mean cessation of employment for Enrolled Nurses, it was made in recognition of the complexities and ambivalence that the profession has experienced since the creation of that particular grade. A number of different proposals were put to the project group which variously suggested that existing Enrolled Nurses should be able to convert their qualification after a minimum period of experience (RCN) whilst other groups felt this to be completely inappropriate. The Project Group, aware of the controversy that this issue had already brought about proposed that the decision about the precise route for conversion should rest with the individual National Boards.

Opportunities for the conversion of Enrolled Nurse qualifications had existed for some time before the publication of *Project 2000, A New Preparation for Practice*. These opportunities had many problems associated with them including cost, the lack of recognition of previous experience and education, and the lack of specific curriculum development for this particular educational activity. In the end the Project Group satisfied itself by proposing that Project 2000 should encompass the need for ensuring:

> The enhancement of opportunities for Enrolled Nurses to enter RGN, RMN, RNMH and RSCN parts of the register (UKCC, 1986, p. 70)

In doing so it recognized the need for the substantial restructuring of the whole of post-qualifying education in the nursing sector.

Project 2000, A New Preparation for Practice is a document of considerable power. The fact that the discussions about its relative merits and shortcomings continue some years after its original publication is testament to that fact. The specific proposals about the development of a new helper grade are, perhaps, scant. There is no doubt, however, that it has played a most significant part in setting the timescale for the re-thinking of the kinds of assistance needed not just by Nurses, but by all the professions involved in the delivery of health care. As well as setting the timescale for change, it has helped to describe the context within which change must take place. Perhaps its most significant contribution is that it is a set of proposals that were developed by an emerging profession, suddenly aware of the need for it to play a major part in providing appropriate contemporary care for its client group.

Many documents, memoranda and circulars have been published since *Project 2000, A New Preparation for Practice* that give a lot of specific detail about the training of Health Care Support Workers and who should be involved in that training. Other chapters in this book will deal with the more useful of these.

Information sources

Birch, J. (1975). *To Nurse or Not to Nurse: An Investigation into the Cause of Withdrawal During Nurse Training*. RCN, London.

Gott, M. (1984). *Learning Nursing: Study of Effectiveness of Relevance to Teaching During Student Nurse Introductory Course*. RCN, London.

HMSO (1972). *Report of the Committee on Nursing. (The Briggs Report)*. HMSO, London.

HMSO (1989). The Nurses, Midwives and Health Visitors (Registered Fever Nurses Amendment Rules and Training Amendment Rules) Approval Order 1989. Statutory Instrument No. 1456. HMSO, London.

Office of Population Censuses and Surveys (1985). General Household Survey. HMSO, London.

Project 2000 Implementation Group (1989). *Nurse Education and Training: Implementation of Project 2000 in 1990–91*. 21st September 1989.

Townsend, P. and Davidson, N. (1982). *Inequalities in Health, The Black Report*. Penguin, London.

UKCC (1986). *Project 2000, A New Preparation for Practice*.

Further information address

United Kingdom Central Council for Nursing, Midwifery and
  Health Visiting,
23, Portland Place,
London,
W1N 3AF.

2

National Vocational Qualification

Introduction

The award of a nationally recognized qualification on successful completion of a training course for the Health Care Support Worker is, to many qualified practitioners who will be involved in the training programmes, still a very grey area. Much has been written about National Vocational Qualifications (NVQs) and what the advantages are to the workforce in the UK. This chapter will explore some of the relevant issues. The National Council for Vocational Qualifications (NCVQ) has produced a vast amount of literature in support of vocational qualifications which may not be generally available to the majority. This literature has been read and inwardly digested and this chapter represents the author's interpretation. There are some terms you need to be familiar with before proceeding to the body of the text. These are described below.

Common terms

Accreditation

The formal act by which the NCVQ simultaneously recognizes statements of competence and awarding bodies and approves qualifications for inclusion within the NVQ framework.

Accreditation of Prior Learning (APL)

The process by which credit is given for prior learning and achievement.

Action plan

As used here, an action plan is a personal statement of actions to be taken in working towards competence.

Area of competence

A sub-division of the total occupational field to which a set of NVQs relate. Normally one set of NVQs, each at different levels, will relate to each area of competence. It is the horizontal sub-division of the total range of employment covered by the NVQ framework.

Assessment

The process of judging the demonstration of an element of competence against a set of specified performance criteria.

Awarding body

A body approved by the NCVQ for the purpose of awarding an NVQ. It may be a single institution or an agreed group of bodies co-operating together for the purposes of offering an NVQ.

Competence

The ability to perform work activities to the standards required in employment.

Prior learning

Previous learning by an individual which has normally not been assessed or certificated.

Standard

The level of performance required for the achievement of an element of competence as indicated by the performance criteria.

Statement of competence

The specification of competence upon which an NVQ is based, stated in the form of the title, units, elements and performance criteria.

Unit (or unit of competence)

A primary sub-division of the competence needed to be achieved for the award of an NVQ, representing a discrete aspect of competence which may be recognized and certificated independently as a credit towards an award. Units comprise one or more elements of competence.

Validating body

An organization which approves programmes delivered by other organizations.

Credit accumulation

The process of certificating and aggregating units of competence over a period of time as a means of achieving the competence needed for an NVQ award. Also applies to other vocational qualifications.

Element (or element of competence)

The smallest part of competence needed to be achieved for the award of an NVQ and sub-division of a unit of competence. Assessment will normally be conducted in respect of each element. An element must be stated with a high degree of precision and will always require performance criteria to indicate the standard at which the element of competence needs to be demonstrated. Elements of competence are comparable with what have been described in other qualification and training systems as competence objectives, learning objectives, learning outcomes or profile statements.)

Experiential learning

The process of acquiring skills, knowledge and understanding through experience. Competence developed through experiential learning can be put forward for accreditation using a variety of forms of evidence.

Level

A vertical sub-division of the NVQ framework used to define progressive degrees of competence according to a generalized system.

National record of vocational achievement (NROVA)

A document or method by which units of competence, certificated by different awarding bodies, may be recorded and accumulated within a common national system.

NVQ criteria

The criteria which awards for accreditation as an NVQ must meet.

NVQ framework

The national system for ordering NVQs according to levels and areas of competence.

Performance criteria

The criteria which indicate the standard of performance required for the successful achievement of an element of competence.

The National Council for Vocational Qualifications

Within the United Kingdom there is a major reform of vocational education underway, which is being directed in England, Wales and Northern Ireland by the National Council for Vocational Qualifications (NCVQ) and in Scotland by the Scottish Vocational Educational Council (SCOTVEC). NCVQ was set up by the Government, following the White Paper *Working Together – Education and Training* (NCVQ, 1986), and set nine specific tasks to achieve, these were to:

(1) Secure standards of occupational competence and to ensure that vocational qualifications are based on them.
(2) Design and implement a new material framework for vocational qualifications.
(3) Approve bodies making accredited awards.
(4) Obtain comprehensive coverage of all occupational sectors.
(5) Secure arrangements for quality assurance.
(6) Set up effective liaison with bodies awarding vocational qualifications.
(7) Establish a national database for vocational qualifications.
(8) Undertake or arrange to be undertaken, research and development to discharge these functions.
(9) Promote vocational education training and qualification.

The White Paper endorsed the recommendations of the *Review of Vocational Qualifications in England and Wales: A report by the working group* (NCVQ, 1986). One of the key elements in this reform is that the individual on a training course will be assessed under normal working conditions, and this will be against the standards set by the occupation/profession. The assessment will in most instances take place in the actual workplace, for example those undertaking a course of training within the National Health Service specifically designed to prepare the Health Care Assistant, would probably undertake the assessment in the wards or departments in the hospital undertaking their training programme, under the supervision of the qualified Nurses. The Nurses involved in the assessment of the Health Care Assistant would also be involved in the coaching and generally helping the student to work towards an NVQ.

NCVQ does not itself issue qualifications but endorses those awarded by examining bodies such as City and Guilds of London Institute (CGLI) or the Business and Technical Education Council (BTEC). Collectively these form the Joint Awarding Bodies.

Vocational qualifications are defined by NCVQ as 'qualifications that relate directly to a person's competence in employment'. When a qualification is formally recognized by NCVQ it is incorporated into the National Vocational Framework and called a National Vocational Qualification (NVQ).

The NCVQ sets about designing the National Vocational Qualifications Framework.

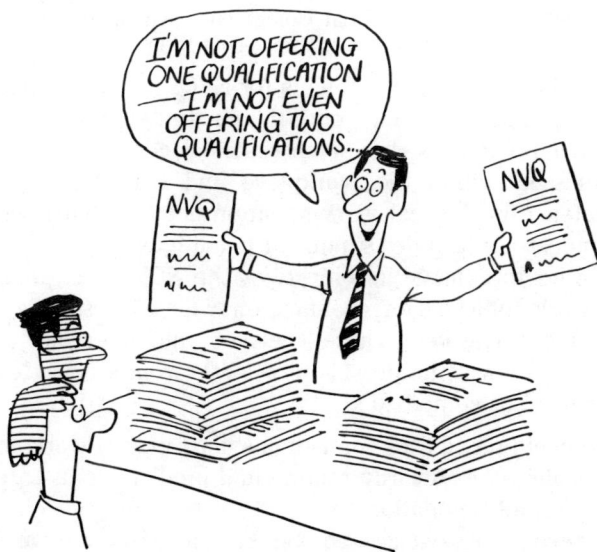

To be part of this framework existing qualifications had to be redesigned to show that they assessed not only the skills and knowledge but also could demonstrate how the skills and knowledge are applied in the work place. In other words the person's ability to do the job, or to use more technical terminology, their *occupational competence.*

One can therefore define an NVQ as a statement of competence which is clearly relevant to the work that is intended to facilitate entry into or progression in employment, further education or training. An NVQ is normally made up of between four and 25 units of competence, the average being between 10 and 15 units. In order to gain the qualification the student is required to demonstrate that he/she is competent within the work situation. In some instances these demonstrations may take place under conditions which realistically simulate the requirement of the work involved. Competence in this context means performing consistently to national standards which are employment led and set by the employers themselves.

> National Vocational Qualifications are not simply statements that a person has achieved certain skills and knowledge, they also indicate that he/she can consistently apply those skills and knowledge in their chosen work area. The holder of an NVQ holds a statement of Occupational Competence which indicates their ability to actually do the job. (Delivering NVQs)

In setting out the requirements for NVQs the NCVQ states that it 'wishes to see the competence demonstrated in the workplace'. It further recognizes that some essential components can only be assessed within the workplace and that 'to demonstrate competence in the real work situation is more demanding than to demonstrate it under simulated conditions'.

In order to achieve its objectives the NCVQ has produced a framework of levels of qualification which is essential to the working of the system. These levels, of which there are four, are intended to cover the provision of NVQs from a basic level to a higher level of competence:

(1) Level I recognizes competence in a range of work activities which are primarily routine and predictable as to provide a broad foundation.

(2) Level II recognizes competence in a broader and more demanding range of work activities involved in greater individual responsibility.

(3) Level III recognizes competence in skilled areas that involve performance at a broad range of work activities including many complex and non routine. Supervisory competence may be required at this level.

(4) Level IV recognizes competence in the performance of complex, technical and professional work activities including supervision and management.

This framework simplifies the structure of vocational qualifications and existing qualifications, with some modification and possible amendment, can in many cases be slotted into the framework and receive NCVQ validation. Providing the criteria set by NCVQ is met then their 'seal of approval' is stamped on it and the qualification receives NVQ status and carries the name of the awarding body, for example BTEC, City and Guilds or Central Council for Education and Training in Social Work (CCETSW).

NVQs are competence-based qualifications 'Statement of Competence' which incorporate the required standards determined by 'The Employer'; who is also responsible for the maintenance of these standards. In order to achieve a competence-based qualification the outputs of education and training must be clearly defined and the standard of performance required clearly stated. This is very important since greater emphasis is placed on performance in employment. Inherent in this is the *assessment* of performance plus assessment of knowledge and understanding which underpins the achievement of a satisfactory level of performance. To aid those involved in the complexity of determining another individual's suitability the NVQ is broken down in such a way as to identify:

(1) The main task area – this is called *a unit of competence*
(2) The unit of competence can be further broken down into smaller task areas which are called *elements of competence*. The points on which you base your judgement or assessment as to whether or not the person could do the task are called *performance criteria*.

For further clarification see Chapter 6 on assessing competence.

The introduction of NVQs heralds a process of change for any organization involved in the provision of programmes enabling individuals to achieve a naturally recognized vocational qualification. In opening up the opportunities for people to gain these qualifications the problem of flexibility had to be addressed. In the literature produced by NCVQ many words were identified as 'Keys' to the practicalities of implementation. Some of these key words are described below.

Competence

There are many different definitions of this – one such is 'the possession and development of sufficient skills, knowledge, appropriate attitudes and experience for successful performance in life roles' which reflects the ability to perform a variety of roles (Further Education Unit, 1984). In respect of NCVQ the notion of vocational competence must include a combination of skill, knowledge, attitudes, plus understanding the tasks involved within a specific occupation. It should also take into account experience. Within the concept of vocational competence *competency* is considered to be an element of the whole. In achieving the elements of competence however small, the individual received *credit*, and these credits can be accrued towards a unit of competence which in turn accumulate towards the award of an NVQ at the relevant level.

Competency does not imply perfection but rather performance at a standard level. This form of assessment responds to the need for flexibility in delivery of education. It could be argued that the provision of competence-based education would lead to the person achieving a series of competences related to a particular job becoming well able to do the job without widening their horizons. However, what the NVQ framework is providing is a system of ladders and bridges by which an individual can progress thus providing the opportunity for further expansion. Some of the opportunities are explored in Chapter 9.

> Underlying the competency-based model is the belief that it is possible to predict and describe competences in some detail prior to their performance. ... from the perspective of purposive action, projects of action are constantly in the making and re-making as their defects and positive aspects become evident. (Grosch, 1987)

This emphasizes the fact that in assessing another individual's ability, ongoing observation is required, and not just a 'one off' view of that individual. The process of development of the individual's performance is as important as the product of the training. If the reasoning behind the required level of performance is to be meaningful to the individual then the learning process should be assessed as well as the learning outcomes. This is particularly relevant in the sphere of caring competencies since many would fail in the objective of ability to do the job if methodology were not incorporated into the assessment of skill outcome.

Within the NVQ framework standards have been set, but are open to subjective interpretation in some instances. Some are more easily standardized than others, for example if one is assessing the competency related to a skill such as typing ability, the criteria may be producing a letter at 50 words per minute with one mistake allowed. In terms of caring skills, however, the determination of competency is open to professional discretion, and more open to a subjective interpretation of the individual's competence. The professional person involved in assessing individuals undertaking the training schemes needs to be both personally and professionally interested, since this process may involve considerable amounts of time. As part of this role, the assessor is required to assess the individual's competence attained in the work situation and document this in the appropriate way in the individual's records towards the qualification.

Credit accumulation

These modules or units are made up of competencies recorded separately in a *record of competence* as *credits* accumulated towards a full *National Vocational Qualification*. The opportunity to acquire these units over a period of time may be an attractive proposition to many who would wish to obtain a vocational qualification. The setting down of competence acquisition in the record of competence, could positively reinforce the learning habit of many who left formal education some time ago and could motivate them to continue their education throughout adult life.

This information will be maintained on a national database for qualifications. Part of this database is a listing of all composite units which make up an NVQ and will be available to anyone who wishes to know what is required to make up an NVQ as a prerequisite to planning programmes of learning. Some elements of the units may have been undertaken in a different form, or the person may be well able to demonstrate competence, in which case this prior learning could be accredited towards the NVQ.

Accreditation of prior learning

NCVQ states 'that with respect to "accreditation of prior learning" that it is not "learning" which is actually being accredited, but the evidence of achievement resulting from learning'. It also states that 'prior achievements are simply those which have occurred in the past'. This learning may have come from independent self-directed study or life experiences drawn from activities other than employment.

What may be required of the individual, in order to be awarded credits towards an NVQ as a result of prior learning, is a demonstration of competence and this may take the form of a test; other evidence may be permissible if deemed to be relevant and up to date. Take for example the person wishing to work in the health care sector in a caring role, who has for the past few years been the sole provider of a 24-hour service of care for a frail elderly parent, or sick child, and who wishes this experience to be credited toward a qualification. It would be reasonable, following a short assessment period within the workplace, to credit this valuable experiential learning towards a qualification. Indeed the person may bring a wealth of knowledge and understanding to caring that others may learn from.

Whilst the NCVQ encourages the development of programmes designed to lead directly to the award for NVQ it also promotes learning in all forms and locations as a continuum of development and updating of individuals. Vocational qualifications have mainly been awarded on completion of a formal programme. Although this traditional route is encouraged, if it were to be the only way to achieve an NVQ the access to qualification would be limited and a wide range of individuals would be debarred from acquiring competence by other means. One of the advantages, therefore, of a credit accumulation system would be the provision of opportunities for more individuals to gain a recognized qualification through different modes of learning, in different locations and content over a variety of timescales. How does this work?

A number of educational establishments throughout the UK are offering distance/open learning programmes which have been validated by an examining body, e.g. BTEC and C & G, for which points are credited towards the certificate which is awarded by them. This is part of the NVQ framework and as such the credits are accrued towards an NVQ.

It is fair to say that although there are obvious advantages of this system there are disadvantages. For instance if the credits are built up over a long period of time there is no guarantee that the knowledge and skill acquired earlier have been retained or are indeed current at the time the NVQ is awarded.

For many individuals the attainment of qualifications is complete before the work-related experience begins. During the course of their working lives these same individuals continue the learning process in the acquisition of new skills and knowledge, and probably at some point will attend courses in relation to their job – but receive no formal recognition for this. Many of the working people have no relevant qualifications to the work they do. That is not to say they do not have the skills and knowledge to do the job but that the system has not allowed for certification of their application of skills and knowledge in their workplace. Take, for example, Auxiliaries within the ward setting. They have an important role within the caring team to fulfil, but their ability to undertake this role is not formally recognized. This is being addressed in many authorities to accredit prior learning so that Auxiliaries will not be disadvantaged in terms of the new 'Support Workers' being introduced into the system, who at the end of their course will have a nationally recognized vocational qualification which provides the opportunity to develop within the role or provides the progression through the levels to acquire an acceptable level for entry into Nurse Education.

To assist those individuals who want to take advantage of obtaining a recognized vocational qualification this flexibility of approach is very important. It does not limit them to undertaking units within a given period of time nor is their choice of unit limited. People can select when, where and how they will accrue their credits. This is as a result of putting the units of learning into packages called '*modules*' which can be 'purchased' by the user when they are ready. The main reason for this is the insistence by the NCVQ that learning should be easily accessible and flexible, and the criteria for the award of an NVQ reflect this by stating:

(1) No restriction to awards by prescribing the form of education and training required, thus learning by any method including prior, experiential, open and distance learning will be acceptable.

(2) No specification of a minimum or maximum period of time in training or work experience before an award can be made.

(3) No upper or lower age limits specified for the assessment and award of a qualification, except where legal constraints make this necessary.

This could lead the way to many of the existing barriers to education and training being removed and those previously disadvantaged being given the opportunity to take advantage. The demographic changes which are highlighting the reduction in the availability of young adults have necessitated this approach in the hope that recruitment and retention of adults can be facilitated.

The unemployed and the female workforce are examples of representative groups for whom this system may present an inviting proposition. This is in keeping with one of the intentions behind this type of programme in that it will broaden the labour market from which employers like the National Health Service draw their staff. It is also hoped that it will attract more men into the 'Support Worker' type role and also more people from ethnic minority groups. The development of the NCVQ framework is not without its implications for Colleges of Further Education. The Colleges have, possibly to a greater extent than other sections of the education system, been aware of the need to provide flexibility of study in order to attract students since there has never been a guarantee that students would attend the courses provided.

Another advantage of this system is the opportunity offered to the individual to 'pick and mix' modules which are appropriate to the role they are undertaking in the workplace and also of interest to them. Therefore the course they follow is tailored to their individual needs. This opportunity is facilitated by those involved in the training who can help the student select and decipher what is relevant at the same time offering guidance and support, and in some instances directing the student along an appropriate pathway to success and achievement.

Information sources

Bennett, T. (1989). *The Assessment of Supervised Work Experience in Higher Education*. Huddersfield Polytechnic.

Education (May 1988). Flavour of the Month. Assessment – the Next Decade.

Further Education Unit (1984). *Towards a Competency-Based System*.

Grosch, P. (1987). *The New Sophists: The Work and Assumptions of the Further Education Unit in Skills and Vocationalism. The Easy Answer*. Open University Press.

Hermann, G.D. (1987). *Competency-Based Vocational Education*. Further Education Unit.

NCVQ. *Its Purposes and Aims*.

NCVQ. *Developing a National System of Credit Accumulation and Transfer*. Information Leaflet No. 1.

NCVQ (1986). *Working Together – Education and Training*.

NCVQ (1987). *A Summary*.

NCVQ (1988). *Introducing National Vocational Qualification for Education and Training*. Information Leaflet No. 2.

NCVQ (1988). *Access and Equal Opportunities in Relation to National Vocational Qualification*. Information Leaflet No. 3.

Open University (1989). *Delivering National Vocational Qualifications – A Guide for Staff Development*.

UDACE (Unit for the Development of Adult Continuing Education) (1990). *An Agenda for Access*.

3

The National Health Service Directorate

Introduction

In April 1991 the existing National Health Service Training Authority (NHSTA) was dissolved and became the National Health Service Directorate responsible to the National Health Service Management Executive. The primary function of this newly formed NHS Directorate Board is to provide a strong link with education and training between the Service and the Management Executive. The Board is representative of the wider world of education and training and as such will give training a higher profile in relation to NHS priority needs and the overall personnel strategies. This new Board will continue to provide the quality of work initiated in its former existence as the NHSTA. Exactly how this will be provided is, at the time of publication of this text, not fully known. However, this Board will still occupy the same address as the NHSTA which is included at the end of this chapter. For the purposes of this particular text it is the work which was initiated and undertaken by the NHSTA which is discussed along with the other bodies involved.

In considering the introduction of a 'new helper' into the health care team the names of various interested 'bodies' have become part of everyday life for those involved in the training and monitoring of this role. Much has been written about the work of these bodies in the various journals and their names have become fairly familiar phrases (Fig. 3.1). The intent of this section is to give some background information as to how they came into being and what they did.

Secretary of State

|

NHSTA

|

Care Sector Consortium (the local industry body)

|

Joint Awarding Bodies

+

Scottish Vocational Educational Council (SCOTVEC)

BTEC	C & G	CCETSW
(Business and Technical Education Council)	(City and Guilds of London Institute)	(Central Council for Education and Training in Social Work)

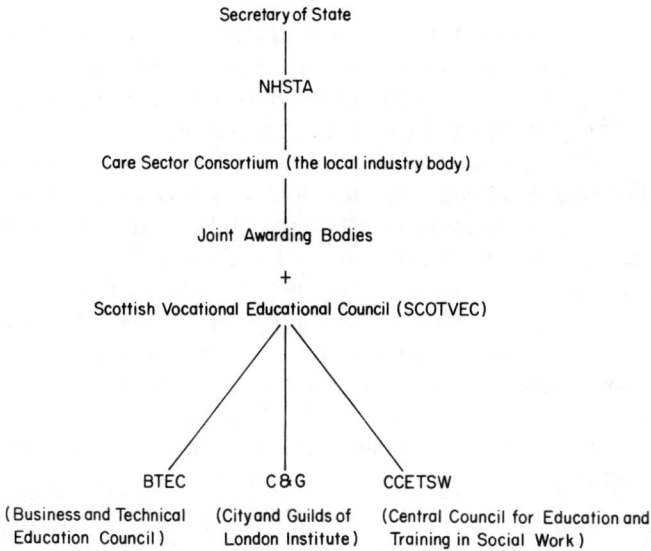

Fig. 3.1. The various interested bodies.

The National Health Service Training Authority (NHSTA)

The NHSTA was established by statutory instrument in 1983. This body was formed by bringing together a number of existing bodies – seven groups were involved in this amalgamation ranging from the Hospital Estate Management and Engineering Centre to the five National Staff Committees covering Nursing, Midwifery and Health Visiting, Ambulance, Estates, Administrative and Clerical and Ancillary Staff. The NHSTA is charged with the performance of functions relating to the training of Officers and Health Authorities under the National Health Service Act 1977. In order to pursue its vast array of functions the NHSTA receives funding via the Department of Health, the Welsh Office, the National Health Service Management Executive and the Training Agency.

When the seven bodies amalgamated, the NHSTA inherited some 200 members of staff, with a wealth of experience, expertise and enthusiasm, from various health-related professions. One of the major elements of the role and function of this newly formed body was the emphasis centred around providing strategic management and support for all those involved in training within the Health Service.

The NHSTA has identified the major purpose of its existence by clarifying and stating its 'mission' which is to 'improve the performance of training in all parts of the NHS in order to support the goals of health care'.

As a means of achieving this mission, the NHSTA has identified *three key purposes*. Firstly, the support of 'change' which is to be facilitated by the training programmes for the NHS Management Executive and Regional General Managers. Secondly the existing learning programmes will be adapted to meet the training needs for training managers in respect of the changes in their future roles. Thirdly the need for a competent workforce is to be provided by developing staff who deliver training and who assess training performance. These are not listed necessarily in order of priority. The NHSTA will implement National Strategies in order to meet priority needs. The resource management needed to meet the priority needs of the Health Service will be met by a supply of training services and agencies set up by the NHSTA.

The main area of work which may be known to people working in health care is the NHSTA's work in relation to 'arranging for a nationally recognized qualification based on agreed standards of performance for managing and delivering health care' or setting up a range of competency-based qualifications for Health Care Assistants. This important role is only part of the NHSTA's remit.

In order to fulfil the need for unqualified personnel responsible for delivering health care, the NHSTA directed the initiation of National and Regional Co-ordinators, who are involved with the local or district co-ordinators responsible for supporting trainers in the work situation. Part of the National and Regional Co-ordinators' role is the dissemination of information from the Secretary of State to the relevant parties. The meetings organized serve to produce an environment which is conducive to the exchange of ideas and experiences in attempts to co-ordinate and formulate strategies for quality training. The NHSTA also produces numerous training packs and programmes designed to help trainers deliver quality programmes of development for staff.

The areas are too varied and numerous to include them all here. Some examples are:

- Training Strategies for Customer Relations Training in the NHS
- Health Pickup – for qualified professionals within the NHS. This is a modular training programme which seeks to improve performance in the workplace by adopting a multidisciplinary approach.

Care Sector Consortium

Health Care Support Worker Project

The Care Sector Consortium was established in October 1988 to develop National Vocational Qualifications (NVQs) for Health Care Assistants and for those working in residential, domiciliary and day care employment.

The project was jointly funded by the Department of Employment Training Agency and the NHSTA, with contributions from other organizations. The NHSTA acted as contractors with lead responsibility for managing the project.

The Consortium is a voluntary body made up of employer and employee representatives from the NHS, Local Government, Voluntary, Private Health, Social Services, United Kingdom Central Council for Nursing, Midwifery and Health Visiting (UKCC), CCETSW, and the Council for the Professions Supplementary to Medicine.

Besides looking at the roles currently filled by the Nursing Auxiliary/Assistant the roles of the Physiotherapy Helper, Occupational Therapy Helper, Speech Therapy Helper, Speech Therapy Assistant, Care Assistants, Foot Care Assistants and Ward Clerks were looked at. It was thought that the potential overlap in some of the competences required of the various role holders warranted joint consideration. Thus it will be seen that the term 'Support Worker' refers to people working within various 'supporting' roles in the Care Sector.

The objectives given to the Care Sector Consortium by the NHSTA were:

(1) To undertake an occupational mapping exercise to define the occupational range and job functions of support workers.

(2) To produce a set of draft national standards competence together with their association performance criteria; identifying those standards of competence which are:
    common to all support workers
    common to some support workers
    specialism.

(3) To identify the essential knowledge and understanding identifying the draft standard of competence.

(4) To check the control of the competences with a representative sample of employment in each of the three areas covered (NHS, Private and Voluntary).

(5) To develop practical and technically sound assessment methods with supporting recording and evaluating systems.

(6) To test draft national standards of competence and assessment methods through a representative pilot study.

(7) To evaluate the pilot study and prepare an implementation plan which includes working with awarding bodies in the development of NVQs which are based on the standards of competence derived from the project.

A study was set up to test the competences when the key role, units and elements had been identified. The field test covered 22 sites across the NHS, Private and Voluntary sectors. This formed the basis of a further pilot study testing the standards of competence to determine their usability for assessment and also testing work-based assessment methods and systems for recording achievement. For the piloting exercise the National Awarding Bodies were involved and would be responsible for awarding NVQs. The report and recommendations were available in early 1990.

Having analysed the draft competences and made recommendations, further developments are to be undertaken. Higher levels of skills will be looked at having developed competences at Levels I and II. Nine qualifications at Level III have been written and it is hoped that these will be made available (at the end of 1990). Assessment was found to be a problem because of the lack of assessors in smaller private and voluntary organizations.

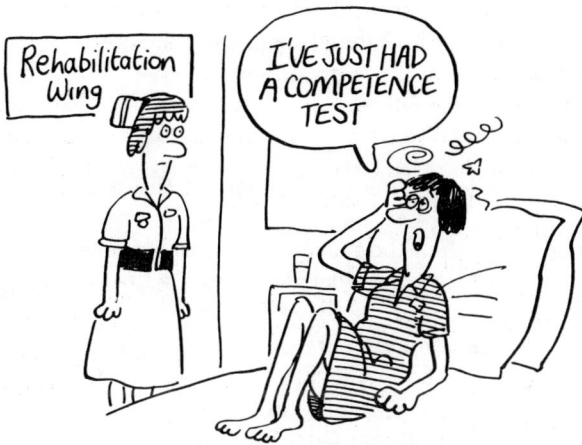

During the development of the Support Worker and Residential and Domiciliary and Day Care (RDDC) projects it was recognized that there were many similarities between the competences developed in the two projects.

Residential, Domiciliary and Day Care Project (RDDC)

When this project was commenced, there was little to help define a national standard within RDDC. The workforce involved in this area number approximately 0.5 million, and have numerous job titles within it. The contract for this undertaking was agreed between the Main Contractor (the Local Government Training Board) and the Training Agency. The project team defined the 'Occupational Domain', that is to say it set about identifying the various roles requiring analysis in order to confirm the validity and reliability of the standards. A distinction was drawn between Social Care and Direct Care. Social Care was defined as a 'generic term' embracing all settings, circumstances were used to describe 'the roles of first hand providers of care'. This included those involved in counselling and advice giving as well as those performing the practical skills involved and associated with care. Employers and employees were included in the organizational framework involved in the care of client groups in a variety of settings. These included RDDC-supported housing and centres for:

- children and their families
- adult people with mental health problems
- adults with learning difficulties
- adults with disabilities
- older people.

It did not include the 'informal' cover, i.e. those with relatives at home.

Having undertaken the research the project team analysed the findings from which there was identified a set of core units which were pertinent to each of the roles identified. The NVQ would be based on this common core plus a prescribed combination of specialized units. The qualification structure is devised with the NCVQ criteria for acceptability in mind.

At present, five National Qualifications are available based on the RDDC and Health Care Assistant (HCA) standards which have been approved by the Care Sector Consortium. A future addition will be new qualifications which are based on an integration of the RDDC and HCA standards which will incorporate appropriate standards related to other sections covered by the Care Sector. The opportunity for those involved in care to gain NVQ is still a very new and exciting venture and as such will be researched fully to identify and plan the most efficient way of offering and implementing the full range of NVQs in the Care Sector.

The NVQs are available through organizations approved by one of the Joint Awarding Bodies, i.e. BTEC, C & G or CCETSW (see Chapter 4). This is provided in agreement with the Care Sector Consortium and the NCVQ in order to provide consistency.

A similar project is underway related to the competence required of those supporting the professionals in the care of the under sevens.

National Occupational Standards

The project to determine and develop a series of employment-led standards of competence which would be credited by NCVQ for Health Care Support Workers was undertaken by the Care Sector Consortium. The result of this work is the production of the National Occupational Standards of competence. These standards are a result of considerable work undertaken related to analysing the role and function of those supporting the work of the health care professionals. Prior to issuing these standards of competence they were tested in England, Scotland and Wales across the range of care settings in both the public and private sectors. In setting the standard, the Care Sector Consortium sought the advice of Nurses, Midwives, Health Visitors, Physiotherapists, Occupational Therapists, Speech Therapists and Chiropodists. The membership of the Steering Group was representative of professional bodies, statutory bodies and awarding bodies together with health care employers and employees.

The project commenced in 1988 funded by the Department of Employment Training Agency and the NHSTA.

The project team was required to establish appropriate standards of competence for those working within support roles in health care which would contribute to the training of the quality of care. In addition to this was the opportunity for these workers to gain access to a nationally recognized qualification at the same time as the opportunity to progress. Determining standards of competence was a complex undertaking, taking into account the various professional disciplines involved in care delivery. Within each discipline, areas were identified which were common to all. These would form the Common Core. There were also areas which were common to some of the roles but not to others and areas which were specialized.

The groupings of the standards are based on NVQ Level I and Level II. In Level I 'Assisting Clients in Care' is made up of 10 units of competence which are required of all Health Care Support Workers. In Level II, 'Direct Personal Care' is made up of 11 units reflecting the standards of competence required of the Health Care Support Worker working mainly in acute settings and 'Enablement Care' is made up of 12 units and is particularly relevant to those where the main focus is on development/rehabilitation.

Many of the core elements of the roles were very similar to those working in settings, e.g. residential. A similar project was looking at competence required for personnel working in day care establishments etc. The National Standards are discussed more fully in Chapter 8.

Integration project

This project was commissioned by the Care Sector Consortium (CSC) in July 1990. It stems from the two earlier projects carried out under the direction of the Consortium. The Residential, Domiciliary and Day Care Project (RDDC), and the Health Care Support Worker Project (HCSW). When both projects reported to the Consortium in May 1990 a large degree of commonality was found to exist, which resulted in a decision to investigate the possibility of integrating the two sets of standards and qualifications.

The integration project is designed to combine the earlier projects to provide consistent, integrated coverage of nationally recognized standards for all occupational groups included in the first two projects. It will also provide a common core foundation for the acquisition of level III NVQs. In effect, this allows for the bringing together of those aspects of work which are common to all, while leaving the distinct areas of work where they arise. The Integration Project has been through a number of phases, resulting in a substantial questionnaire containing the proposed NVQs and Scottish Vocational Qualifications (SVQs) and the standards on which they are based. This questionnaire has been widely distributed to key interest groups. In some instances a pilot will be undertaken in a number of 'integrated sites' where health authorities, private sector and local authorities will 'test' the work in practical situations.

Information sources

NHSTA. *Update on Health Care Assistant Training.*
NHSTA (1989). *Support Worker Project – Pilot Stage.*
NHSTA. *Health Care Credit System – A Guidance Note for External Verifiers.*
NHSTA. *Youth Training Good Practice Guide.*
NHSTA. *Purpose, Activities and Use of Funds.*
Further Education Unit. *Support YTS.*

Further information address

NHSTA (National H.S. Directorate),
St Bartholomews Court,
Christmas Street,
Bristol,
BS1 5BT.

4

Joint Awarding Bodies

Within the framework of vocational qualifications there are, as stated in previous chapters, a number of awarding bodies involved in the National Vocational Framework. In this chapter the intention is to try and explain some of the grey areas and to show how one of these bodies links with the National Council for Vocational Qualifications (NCVQ) framework. The choice does not infer preference on the part of the author but the body chosen is somewhat more familiar than the others. The one chosen to explore is the Business and Technical Education Council (BTEC). BTEC was established by the Department of Education and Science and given the role and function of the promotion and development of high-quality courses which were closely related to a variety of work areas, for example working within the health care sector.

The Business and Technical Education Council (BTEC)

BTEC is a self financing, independent body offering a vast range of courses covering a wide range of subjects. In order that an establishment can undertake the running of a course leading to a BTEC qualification it has to receive approval. Courses are normally undertaken in Colleges of Further and Higher Education or Polytechnics and successful course participants receive a qualification which is recognized by employers, professional bodies and educationalists throughout the United Kingdom. The income which BTEC receives from the fees paid by course members is used to enable BTEC to monitor and evaluate the existing courses and improve where necessary and also to approve, monitor and evaluate new courses. By doing so, more and more courses are evolving to meet the needs of an ever-changing society.

Before approving an establishment to run a course which carries the BTEC seal of approval, the establishment applying to run the course has to prove to BTEC that it has the appropriate resources available and the necessary staff, expertise and equipment which are required to conduct a high quality course successfully. An important part of the formulation of the syllabus for these courses is the involvement of the employers. This is an important part of the work of BTEC in that the courses are work-related courses and employers are obviously keen that people who are undertaking a BTEC course in order to enter employment are receiving appropriate instruction and experience. In recent months a number of Colleges of Nursing have applied to BTEC to become approved centres for running BTEC courses designed to prepare their Health Care Assistants.

The BTEC courses can be studied by people who are already in full-time education or on a day release basis for those in employment. They are also available to be taken at evening classes or as part of an open learning programme. The courses, since they are work-related courses, are a combination of theory and practice so that employers can be sure that someone with a BTEC qualification as well as being able to write about the job actually knows how to do it. People undertaking a course are encouraged to find out certain information for themselves and to develop skills in communication and working within a team. Because of the approach to the courses people undertaking them are assessed by a variety of methods, and because of the different methods employed the course participants develop the ability to work on their own initiative as well as part of a team. Many of the courses provided, including those related to health care, include work experience placements. All the activities undertaken as part of the course are intended to help the learner to discover what they are good at and to build upon these strengths and also to further develop those areas where improvement is necessary and by doing so help to increase their confidence in themselves.

Within the BTEC framework itself there are two main types

of BTEC qualification, i.e. certificates and diplomas. Both the certificate and the diploma courses are available at each of the levels in BTEC of which there are three:

- First,
- National
- Higher National.

Certificate courses are usually studied on a part-time basis whereas the diploma courses are normally full time, although they can be studied on a part-time basis but the completion time is longer. The standard of both the certificate and diploma courses at each of the levels is the same, but the diploma course covers a much broader range of subjects. This is to give the full-time student a wider introduction to career opportunities. The length of the courses available ranges from 1 to 3 years depending on the level and whether it is a certificate or diploma course.

A BTEC course is made up of units which are both theoretical and practical in nature and contain in most instances 'core' and 'optional' subjects. The core subjects are compulsory and are intended to develop essential knowledge and skills with the optional subjects chosen by the person undertaking the course. The choice of option is varied but all colleges do not offer all choices, the learner chooses the areas in which they are interested or that are appropriate to the area of work in which they would like to be involved. Each unit of a BTEC course is graded separately as a pass, merit or distinction.

There are over 250 BTEC courses to choose from and at any time there are over 0.5 million people enrolled on them in approved institutions throughout the United Kingdom. The people who enrol on these courses range from the school leaver joining the full-time courses, to adults joining the part-time courses. Many of these people who enrol for the part-time courses are doing so in order to improve their skills and knowledge for promotion purposes within their chosen area of work. There are of course those people who have been absent from work for a variety of reasons who may consider undertaking a BTEC course prior to returning to work, or those who choose to change their careers and complete BTEC courses as a means of learning new skills. The courses available are open to anyone who wishes to undertake them and can meet the entry requirements set by BTEC.

The cost of courses varies and is usually free to full-time students under the age of 18 years of age. Those people enrolling on the Higher National courses in most instances have their fees paid by the Local Education Authority and receive a grant. Employed people undertaking part-time courses as part of their employer's requirements usually have their fees paid by the employer. There are available to people who are unemployed, schemes sponsored by the Employment Training Agencies for which they receive the appropriate allowance from the Training Agency whilst undertaking the course which on successful completion could lead to full-time employment. An example of this type of course offered is the Health Care Assistant training course. Although as part of a course of this nature the person would be required to work within the clinical areas they would not be paid a salary, but prospects for employed status are usually open to the successful course participant who could, with appropriate advice and support, continue their studies to an appropriate level which would be acceptable for entry to professional education. There are also available a range of continuing education courses and BTEC together with City and Guilds offers the Certificate in Pre-Vocational Education (CPVE) and foundation courses.

It is generally recognized that the qualifications awarded by BTEC have appropriate status with the more generally accepted academic qualifications for example BTEC Higher National Awards are regarded as and normally accepted as approaching degree standard. BTEC National Awards are accepted as equivalent to 'A' level standard and BTEC First Awards are accepted as 'GCSE' standard. Together with other awarding bodies BTEC is working with the NCVQ (see Chapter 2) to ensure that the awards made fit into the National Framework.

The BTEC First Course in Caring

This course is primarily designed for people who wish to pursue a career in the caring services within either the Public or Private Sector. Those who enrol for such a course may be school leavers, people already working within the health care sector or unemployed people seeking to train for a role within the health authorities as Health Care Assistants or as a first step toward professional education. The course aim is to develop appropriate knowledge and skill required in order to help care for people in a variety of health care settings who present with a variety of problems. For entry to this course the prospective student does not normally require formal educational qualifications such as GCSEs but some establishments may ask for them. Candidates must be 16 years old or over and should have attained a level of education which would enable them to cope with the demands of the course. The students undertaking this course are prepared for a wide range of jobs within the health care sector including Care Assistants in residential establishments, Health Care Assistants, Nursery Assistants and Physiotherapy Assistants.

The course is composed of three compulsory, or core, components plus a selection of optional units.

Core components

Common skills

This aims to enable the student to develop a broad spectrum of general skills including communication skills, working in a team with others, problem solving and planning and organizing. These areas are all related to the area of work in which the student is employed.

Behavioural and community studies

This encourages the student to look at society as a whole and the effects society has on the development of the individual. It also incorporates an identification of the needs of different sections of the community and of the services provided in an attempt to meet these needs.

Data collection

This helps the student develop the ability to use information technology in the collection of data relevant to the work he or she is undertaking and, when the information is collected, in its analysis.

Optional units

There is a wide range of optional units available for the student to undertake, but all colleges do not offer all choices or the same options. The kind of units available to students may include biology, caring skills, first aid, health education and human development.

Another important feature of this course is the range of placements available for the student which may include hospitals, day nurseries, schools and voluntary organizations. In assessing the student on this course the methods employed are varied and designed to develop the student's own ability in different areas and may include assignments, project work, case studies, practical exercises and written examinations. For example, a student may be asked to complete a course assignment related to the provision of services for the elderly or mentally ill within the community. The student, with the support of his or her tutor, would set about determining the sources from which to obtain the relevant information and once this is decided would carry out an investigation, the result of which would be fed back to the student's peer group on the course, and also perhaps to the managers for whom the student is working. In undertaking this form of assessment the student is utilizing a number of skills and demonstrating his or her progress in their development.

As stated earlier in the chapter, the BTEC First Certificate courses normally take 1 year to complete on a part-time basis with the first diploma courses taking 1 year full time and 2 years part time to complete. Some establishments may introduce students to the format of study on a first certificate course and offer in the second year, to those who express an interest, the additional units to convert the certificate to a diploma. Successful completion of the First Certificate/Diploma courses qualifies the student for entry to related BTEC National Courses.

BTEC National courses in health studies

As with the First Certificate/Diploma course these courses are designed for people who wish to work within the health care sector or are already employed and wish to take the opportunity to study on the type of course with a view to advancing within their chosen area of work. The difference between this course and the BTEC First course is the level at which it is maintained and also the entry requirements. In order to be eligible to undertake a National course the prospective student must be 16 years old or over and possess a BTEC First award in a relevant area, or four GCSEs at grade 'C' or above, or appropriate qualifications which are acceptable (your local College of Further Education will be able to supply details). The course follows the same kind of pattern as the BTEC First in that there are core and optional units.

Core units

These are:

Basic Applied Science
Human Physiology
Social Development
Data Interpretation and Investigation
Community Assignment.

Optional units

These may include:

Applied Biological Science
Applied Human Physiology
Physiology
Behavioural Science
Biochemistry
Chemistry
Health and the Environment
Health Education

This course, like the BTEC First course, offers a variety of work related placements for the student.

After completing a BTEC National Certificate/Diploma course in health studies some students may wish to continue their studies. For example those who have completed the Certificate course may wish to 'convert' this to a Diploma and carry on with the required units in order to do this. Those who have completed the National Diploma may wish to enter Professional Education in one of the health care areas such as Nursing, Physiotherapy, Social Work or Speech Therapy.

The student may, of course wish to continue in full-time education and indeed may enter a course of study leading to a degree.

Levels of courses

BTEC First Certificates and Diplomas

These are normally taken by school leavers who have chosen the general area of work they wish to enter.

The Diploma takes 1 year full time or 2 years part time. The Certificate takes 1 year on a part-time basis. BTEC has no formal entry requirements, but some colleges prefer GCSEs. First qualifications lead on to employment, or to BTEC National courses.

BTEC National Certificates and Diplomas

These are for junior managers or administrators and technicians. The Diploma takes 2 years full time or 3 years part time. The Certificate takes 2 years part time. Entry requirements are:

- a BTEC First Certificate or Diploma, or
- four GCSEs at grade 'C' or above, or
- certain other qualifications, such as a Certificate in Prevocational Education (CPVE) with a suitable profile.

BTEC National qualifications lead on to employment or to higher education. Some students go on to BTEC Higher National courses. Others, expecting to obtain the grades required by Polytechnics and Universities, apply for degree courses.

BTEC Higher National Certificates and Diplomas

These qualify people to work at managerial, supervisory and higher technician level. The Diploma takes 2 years full time or 3 years part time. The Certificate takes 2 years part time. Entry requirements are:

- a BTEC National Certificate or Diploma, or
- at least one A level and supporting GCSEs at grade 'C' or above.

Holders of BTEC Higher National qualifications can often be admitted to the second or third year of a degree course in a related subject.

BTEC can be seen as an alternative route of entry to Further or Higher Education.

City and Guilds of London Institute

This is probably the most familiar of the Joint Awarding Bodies since it has been in existence and operational for over 100 years. This body operates under the auspices of a Royal Charter which has determined that the role and function of City and Guilds is the advancement of technical and scientific education. This service is provided for the individual, industry and commerce and the Public Sector services. In many respects City and Guilds and BTEC are organized in the same manner. As with BTEC, City and Guilds is a self-financing organization without political affiliation. During the span of its existence and activities the organization has developed considerable experience and expertise in all facets of the educational process. Along with the Central Council for Education and Training in Social Work (CCETSW) and BTEC this expertise and experience is being pooled to advantage those people who wish to accrue units of competence towards a National Vocational Qualification (NVQ). City and Guilds is involved in the identification of requirements in terms of both education and training which are perceived as necessary by both industry and the individual consumer. Having identified the need City and Guilds will design schemes which will meet the identified needs and design appropriate assessment and evaluation strategies. Successful completion leads to the award of the City and Guilds certificate which is a recognition of the competence of the successful individual.

The range of customers for City and Guilds courses is extensive ranging from 14 to 16 year olds undertaking courses leading to basic skill awards, foundation awards and vocational preparation awards, through the 16–21 year old bracket, who may be full-time or part-time students or those on Youth Training (YT) schemes undertaking courses leading to Certificates in Pre-Vocational Education or specific vocational awards, through to mature individuals who are seeking vocational qualifications, such as those embarking on courses for Health Care Support Worker roles or skills training in order to progress within their chosen jobs, or seeking a different job. These individuals may be undertaking such courses which would lead to Special Vocational Awards career extension and first-level management awards or Technical Teacher/Trainer awards for example City and Guilds 730 – Further Education Teachers Certificate, which many clinical nurses have undertaken.

City and Guilds also provide opportunities for people of all ages who wish to pursue schemes related to leisure or recreational activities. As with the other members of the Joint Awarding Bodies, City and Guilds is co-operating with the National Council for Vocational Qualifications (NCVQ) to support the NVQ framework and as such is increasing the flexibility and availability of its services through a credit transfer system.

City and Guilds courses

As with BTEC, the City and Guilds London Institute provides appropriate courses for intending Health Care Assistants for example '356 Practical Caring Skills' and '331 Family and Community Care'. These courses, as with BTEC, could be credited towards a National Vocational qualification. They may be undertaken at local Colleges of Further Education or a College of Nursing or as a combined venture.

The course on Family and Community Care (C & G 331) does not require the candidate to have formal qualifications but they must be 16 years of age or over and have completed 5 years of secondary education to enter the first year of this 2-year course. Mature students are considered on an individual basis and may, if they have relevant training and experience, be admitted to the second year of the course.

The minimum age for entry to the second year is 17 years of age. The course is intended to develop within the individual a

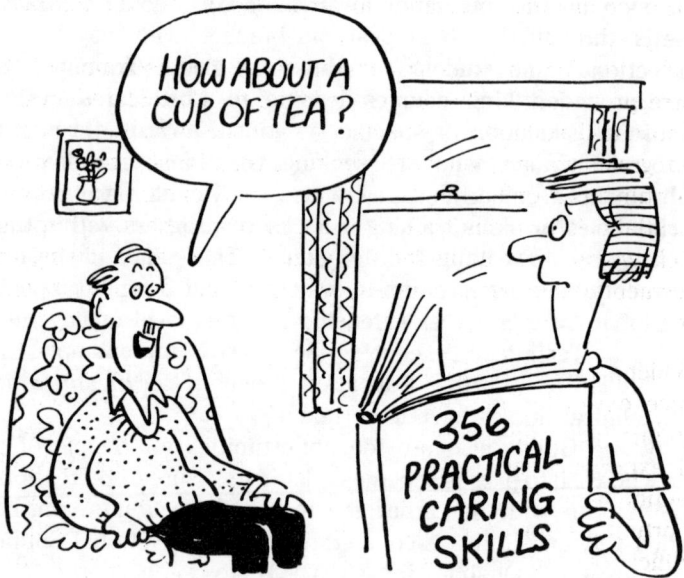

range of skills and knowledge related to the role of care workers and includes areas of study such as communication skills and practical skills. The course participant will also be involved in the acquisition of knowledge and skills in relation to welfare services social groupings and issues relating to the multicultural society. As part of the course the participant will be able to experience a range of placements in which they, under supervision, can apply the theory to the practical situation in relation to working with clients and colleagues.

Practical Caring Skills (356)

This particular course is designed to encourage an awareness of the relevant attitudes, skills and knowledge that are required in a caring situation, and also to allow the student the opportunity to experience a variety of care settings following which the student would be able to make informed choices as to his or her particular interests and possible career pathways in health care. The course covers aspects of development of the individual throughout life and gives details of the range of services available to the community and the different groups which make up society.

Selection for entry to this course is at the discretion of the centre providing it. This course may be of particular relevance to those undertaking YT. The structure of the course is such that it integrates the various components of the course, and provides opportunities for placements in a wide variety of caring situations. Essentially it is intended to be a 'practical' orientated course which would draw upon the individual's experience during the placements in order to provide for significant learning to take place.

Whichever course is available locally or is preferred (if a choice exists for the individual) the benefits of introducing a system which takes into account the existing skills, knowledge and experience of the individual must be a step in the right direction. One of the benefits of this system is the provision of opportunities for individuals who do not possess recognized qualifications to enter a course of preparation and gain a nationally recognized qualification, as well as the opportunity for progression along a clearer career pathway (see Chapter 9).

On an individual basis, recognition is made that a student's experience in both previous employment and indeed life itself is meaningful and can be utilized to the mutual benefit of both peers on the course and the clients with whom they are involved. This surely is a way of instilling national pride, to whatever degree, and also gives the student a sense of purpose. There is the opportunity for the individual to move on to bigger and better things!

The Central Council for Education and Training in Social Work (CCETSW)

This body forms the third member of the Joint Awarding Bodies, and is the body primarily concerned with the monitoring and approval of courses leading to qualifications in social work. CCETSW was established in 1971 and since 1983 has been responsible for the development of training for social workers approved to carry out statutory duties under Mental Health Legislation. Since 1986 CCETSW has been responsible for approving training programmes run by local authorities. This type of programme is available for those wishing to work within this area of care but not necessarily a course leading to qualification as a Social Worker. One such course is the Preliminary Certificate in Social Care. This course is aimed at those people who wish to work in social or health care services. This is a 2-year course in which CCETSW does not require formal academic qualification as a means of entry, but does require the potential student to be able to work to, and cope with, the GCSE work of the course. As part of this course the student has the opportunity to study for a variety of GCSEs or 'A' levels but this is the individual's choice. Other qualifications awarded are in relation to work experience and are vocational qualification orientated. An interesting part of the course involves students spending a week away from home on outdoor pursuits. To undertake this course there is no specified age limit, and quite a proportion of potential students are mature students.

During the 2 years, the student has the opportunity to undertake workplace experience in a variety of settings including hospital wards, working with mentally and physically handicapped people, the elderly and children. During the first year this is normally for 1 day per week, increasing to 2 days during the second year. Successful completion of a course of this nature enables the individual to seek employment in a variety of care settings including children's and elderly persons' homes or can lead to further training, for example in social work.

Information sources

BTEC. *Assessment and Grading.*
BTEC. *Handbook for Moderators.*
BTEC. *Recognition of BTEC Awards.*
City and Guilds. *The Next Five Years* (1988–1993).
City and Guilds (1990). *Introduction of NVQs in Social and Health Care.*
Dept Education & Science (1989). *Courses Leading to the BTEC First Certificate Award: A Report by H.M. Inspectorate.*

Further information addresses

BTEC,
Head Office,
Central House,
Upper Woburn Place,
London.

City and Guilds of London Institute,
76, Portland Place,
London, W1N 4AA.

CCETSW,
Derbyshire House,
St Chad's Street,
London,
WC1H 8AD.

5

Training and Enterprise Councils (TECs)

Training & Enterprise Councils (TECs) are being formed in an attempt to restructure the approach to training and enterprise development within the United Kingdom. The task of the TECs is to develop the quality and effectiveness of training and business assistance programmes which were run prior to their formation by the Employment Training (ET) and Youth Training Schemes (YTS). Eventually the TEC will function as a catalyst for change by serving as a forum where economic and social needs are assessed within the Authority. The TEC will be an independent company whose Boards of Directors will be drawn from employers in the Private Sector, leaders in education voluntary organizations and the Public Sector. It provides the opportunity to restructure the approach to enterprise and training through human development. Essentially the principles underlying these changes will shape the nature of the TEC.

Today's local labour markets demand flexibility and innovation in meeting their specific needs in relation to training. In meeting these needs within a broad national framework the adoption of employer-led partnerships would be advantageous – this fits in with the National Council for Vocational Qualifications (NCVQ) framework of qualifications and training programmes to achieve them.

Opportunities for young persons

The aim of the Government in relation to opportunities for the young is that they should have access to education or training which would enable them to attain a vocational qualification and also to obtain employment. TECs will help the Government in the achievement of their desired state by helping to smooth the transition from education to employment. TECs will endeavour to contract sufficient places as training schemes in order to meet the Government's guarantee of an offer of YTS places for every young person. As part of its role, the TEC may tailor some of the existing schemes and where required be involved in the development of new initiatives, in an attempt to expand opportunities for flexible work or study. An important aspect of the work of the TEC in relation to youth training is the continuation of moves towards improving the links between education provision and the business community. Some of these links are already well established and the TEC is working closely with them to support their activities on either a formal or informal basis. TECs are aiming to achieve an appropriate and coherent approach which recognizes the many sources of support for schools and new opportunities for young people which will enable them to achieve the employment requirements of the 1990s in terms of skill, competence and qualification.

Another major area in which the TEC is involved is in enabling unemployed people to attain skills which are required for the job market by planning and delivering ET in keeping with the requirements of local employers. This will involve the creation of opportunities for those groups of unemployed people previously barred from employment for a variety of reasons. Linked with this will be the design of opportunities for women, older workers and newly unemployed people to equip them adequately to re-enter the job market. By involving itself in this venture the accessibility, quality and relevance to ET will be improved.

TECs will market the importance of training as a business strategy and an investment rather than an optional cost, and thus provide a system of 'training through life'. The actual upgrading of skill or 're-skilling' is primarily the responsibility of the employer with the TEC in an advisory role, enhancing access to information. It is also useful to note that involvement of the TEC by groups of employers sharing a common interest could lead to a collective investment which would prove more cost effective and also improve the flexibility of the methodology adopted for training. By utilizing the resources of ET, YTS and others, the

TECs will be instrumental in the design of customized programmes of training in the preparation of a skilled workforce for occupations where there is a skill shortage.

How will the TEC work?

Each TEC is required to produce a 'Business Plan' which will express its vision, and role within its own particular community. This plan will also include the strategy for meeting the needs identified and also describes the local economic and social characteristics set against both national and international trends in terms of skill deficit. The plan will demonstrate achievable goals at the same time ensuring equal opportunities and health and safety training for those undertaking the various training schemes. This plan is developed on a rolling basis over 3 years which will include annual budgets and operational targets.

The TECs will link with each part of the community: Private Sector employers, Local Authorities, Health Authorities, Voluntary Organizations, Trade Unions, parents, trainees and those people with entrepreneurial flair wishing to set up small businesses.

In 1989 the National Training Task Force (NTTF) was established as an advisory body to the Secretary of State for Employment and also to assist in the carrying out of this training responsibility throughout Great Britain.

One of the principal aims of this body is to ensure that the TECs, when fully established, meet the requirements required in terms of standards of excellence and the provision of high-quality programmes. The TECs will provide a unique opportunity to mould and develop training and enterprise systems during the 1990s. The decision taken to address positively the provision of means to achieve recognized skills and qualification, determined as a requirement by employers, is not the easy option but is the vision of a more enterprising and skilled workforce of the future. This option, to succeed, must draw upon all the resources available within the community and therefore will contribute to the economic growth and development of the community in which the TECs are based.

Employment Training (ET) was launched in 1988, and since

then the records of achievement have been remarkable. Over 400 000 people have joined ET to take advantage of the wide range of training schemes offered by a variety of companies. It is fair to say the ET is the largest and most successful adult training programme to be introduced in this country. The range of training programmes made possible by ET is expanding and represents a massive investment in equipping those who join the scheme with the skills required of the workforce as we move into the 1990s.

What is ET?

The fundamental idea behind ET is really quite simple. It is about offering and providing people with the skills required by employers in an attempt to help them to resolve their skill-shortage problems. The training period is normally up to 1 year in duration and is a combination of theory and related practice which, where possible, leads to the award of a vocational qualification (see Chapters 4 and 5). Essentially ET is a partnership between the Government, the employers and the people who wish to improve their career prospects. The scheme offers the prospective employers the opportunity to be involved in the training of their

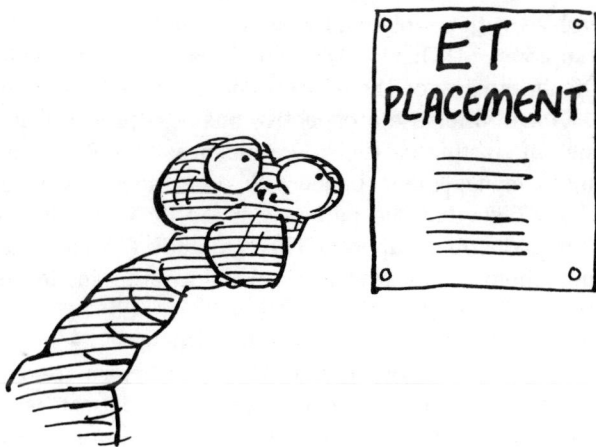

potential workforce. In order for this to be realized, employers provide work experience placements to those on the training courses in order to meet needs which have been specifically identified. This linking of related theory to actual practice affords the trainee the opportunity to gain a high-quality training in preparation for the increasing number of jobs which are becoming available. The partnership approach to ET is very evident in the inner-city areas where the quality of the training schemes is very important to the range of options available to meet specifically identified needs. In urban areas the schemes are made more relevant and are also strengthened by the support and sponsorship of local organizations. ET provides training across a wide range of occupations including schemes devised to provide the opportunity for people to enter the caring professions as Health Care Assistants. Training is provided in a variety of establishments for the range of schemes available, including Colleges of Nursing, Universities, and Colleges of Further Education.

A major feature of ET is local planning and local delivery, thus making sure that the people who are training are undertaking schemes which prepare them for the kinds of jobs available in their communities. ET also has programmes designed specifically to help people with special needs including practical help for those with disabilities, those people who are returning to work following a long absence, people whose first language is not English and those who need initial training in basic skills. ET is also involved with people who wish to branch out into the world of self employment. This kind of venture can be a very challenging and difficult experience therefore preparation for this major step is vital. ET can offer the prospective business person training in the basics of starting up their own business and also in aspects of business management. Links with other agencies have been forged by ET so that the person starting up in small business can receive ongoing support. This expanding area is already attracting sponsorship in the form of awards made to new ventures.

To undertake any of the ET training schemes does not incur any cost on the part of the trainee. The programmes are designed primarily for unemployed people who are out of work for whatever reason for a period of 6 months or more. However, under certain circumstances, others may be eligible who have been unemployed for a shorter period of time. Once accepted on to one of the training programmes they receive their full benefit in the normal way. In addition to this the trainee receives a training allowance with excess travel costs over a specified amount being met by ET. In some instances the trainee may qualify for a bonus payment on completion of the training programme.

How do people join ET?

The answer is really quite simple, if the person is aged between 18 years of age and 60 years of age and has been unemployed for 6 months or more he or she is normally eligible to join ET. The 6-month period of unemployment can include:

- Signing on at an Unemployment Benefit Office.
- Receiving incapacity benefits such as Invalidity Benefit, Sickness Benefit or Severe Disablement Allowance.
- Receiving Income Support as a lone parent where the youngest child is in full-time education.
- If your partner is claiming benefit for you as a dependant and satisfies the rules.
- Time spent on a custodial sentence may also count towards the 6 months. There are, within the rules pertaining to eligibility to join ET courses, contingencies made for those returning to the labour market following a break for domestic reasons and ex-regular members of HM Forces.

A variety of referral routes to these schemes are available through Job Centres, restart interviews or by contacting the Training Agency.

Who are the Training Agents and what do they do?

For most people wishing to take advantage of the schemes offered, the Training Agents will be the initial point of entry to ET. The Training Agent will assist people to assess their training needs and also explore with them the available training opportunities. This process will involve the identification and recording of the client's previous learning and experience and provision of information about opportunities in employment. As part of its advisory role the Training Agency will give the clients information regarding vocational education opportunities. On the basis of the meeting between the client and the Training Agency, they will produce together an individual 'action plan' which will take into account the identified areas of strengths and weaknesses and provide a broad outline of training. Once the action plan is devised the Training Agency will match the client with appropriate Training Managers.

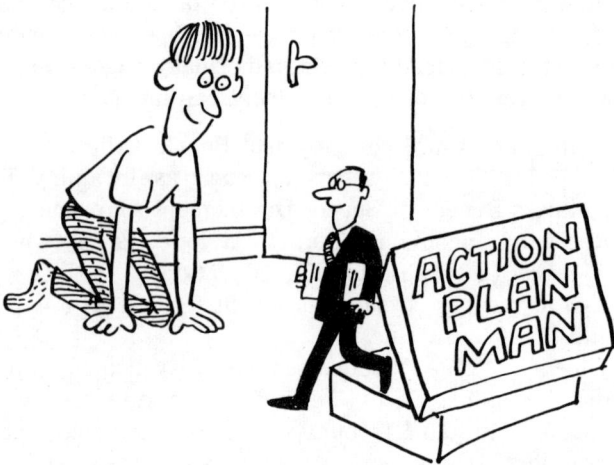

Training Managers

Training Managers are the approved employers who will provide the necessary training. This training will be a mix and match of theory and practice designed to meet the needs of the individual. As part of this plan, training will be the acquisition of recognized vocational qualifications awarded by one of the validating bodies linked to the National Vocational Framework. The skill development offered by the Training Managers may be a fairly broad spectrum or specialized skill related to a particular occupation. For example, some Health Authorities will offer a wide range of skills to those wishing to work in a supportive role in nursing or non-nursing. This would involve a set of core skills appropriate to all with special options for the area in which the individual will gain practical skills. Employer involvement in this process is vital to ET being successful. The involvement of the employers might be as Training Agents, Training Managers, practical training providers, project sponsors or project hosts.

Within the framework of ET is a service available to Training Managers and Training Agents providing assistance and advice in matters concerning clients with special needs. This is called the Employment Rehabilitation Service (ERS). The Training Agents/Managers may refer to this service clients whose condition needs further investigation or those where difficulty may be encountered in the implementation of the initial action plan. For example, it may include those people with disabilities either physical or mental, as with learning difficulties.

In all schemes provided by ET initiatives a high-quality training is assured in terms of design content and delivery. In this undertaking Training Agents and Training Managers are required to secure approval against a set of criteria. Part of the role in the assurance of the quality of the training programmes is making sure that all those involved with the programme understand what is required. It is necessary for the trainers to be able to demonstrate how the parts of the programme combine to produce the desired outcomes and how achievement of competence is demonstrated with a system of progression and accreditation towards a vocational qualification where appropriate.

Essentially ET is about helping unemployed people acquire and develop the skills and knowledge required to compete in the employment market. Prior to undertaking ET programmes they may have been 'put off' applying in response to job advertisements such as 'Recent experience in this area of work essential' or 'Must have recognized qualification'.

The programmes provided under the ET scheme address these issues and also involve many organizations and prospective employers who provide the 'on the job' training. Equally, as well as benefiting the person who embarks on a programme, the employers can reap rewards from their valuable contribution to the schemes in that they have greater access to people who are motivated and want to develop skills. This is evident since ET is a voluntary programme. Another benefit to the employer is the development of an alternative route for recruitment through training schemes, advantageous in that the numbers of school leavers available is diminishing. Because of the involvement of the employers in the design and development of the programmes they can be certain that they have access to skilled people who have undertaken a course which equips them to meet the employers' requirement. This also gives the employer the opportunity to get to know the individuals and assess their potential before having to make a firm commitment to employ on a permanent basis.

Youth Training

In 1989 the Government announced the significant changes 1990 would bring to the opportunities available in the training for young people. The existing Youth Training Scheme (YTS) courses are being redesigned to incorporate a more flexible approach to learning and also to give young people the chance to acquire nationally recognized qualifications and improve their prospects in the labour market. This scheme will be known as Youth Training (YT) and is available to all young people, with the exception of students looking for employment during holidays, overseas students subject to employment restrictions, young people who have done or are doing ET courses and those still at school. If the person is under 18 years of age and not in employment but is seeking work, there is a guarantee of a place on YT. This service is managed by locally based TECs who designed relevant courses in conjunction with the employers in order to provide opportunities to meet local employment demands. For the young people presently undertaking YTS programmes the opportunity to complete the course is there, but the offer of entering a YT course may be available, for example depending on the length of the YTS course and how long the individual has to complete the course, an offer may be made to transfer to YT. The individual then has the option of remaining on YTS or transferring to YT. The YT programme includes a variety of learning modes so the individual has the opportunity to select the most appropriate option which best suits their particular circumstances. This approach affords the individual a choice, even if not sure of career direction, and it also provides a good start on the career ladder. The programmes vary in length dependent on what the individual is attempting to achieve. Those young people in employment undertaking a YT programme will still get a full wage, those unemployed undertaking YT programmes will receive a training allowance, which in some instances may be 'topped up' by the placement employer.

In relation to the NHS, the Price Waterhouse Report 'Feasibility Study into YTS in Health and Social Care Programmes' strongly favoured this type of scheme and saw it as a means of providing a 'high quality training' for those in a support role.

The trends today show a decline in the 16–19 year old age group which will accelerate over the next 5 years. Along with other employers, the NHS may face a short range of recruits with the qualifications required to enter professional education. As a potential employer the attraction of young people is important. The YT programme provides the NHS with appropriate young people working towards acquiring relevant skills and recognized qualifications, at the same time affording the Health Service a young workforce which has experience of health-care related work during training programmes. YT will provide another strand in recruitment of possible health care workers and fits in

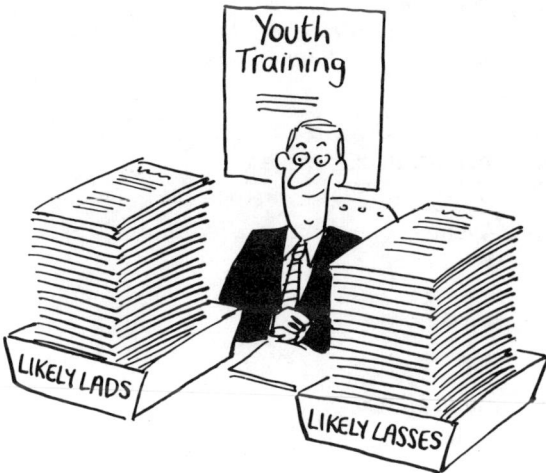

well with other schemes designed to create opportunities such as ET. The schemes are a means of giving those who wish to take advantage of the offer the opportunity to acquire skills and knowledge, along with a nationally recognized qualification. It also provides a structured approach to career prospects and, as such, opens up a new and exciting future.

Information sources

DHSS (1987). *The Role and Preparation of Support Workers to Nurses, Midwives and Health Visitors and the Implications for Manpower Service Planning.*
The Training Agency
    ET. The Facts.
    Employment Training for Women.
    ET. A General Guide to Employment Training, Eligibility and Allowances on Employment Training.
    ET. It's Your Future – Shape It.
       Training Manager Prospectus.
       How ET can Change and Shape your Future Workforce.
       Continuing Assessment and Recording Achievement No. 5.
    TECs – A Guide to Planning.
    ET in the Health Care Sector.
Further Education Unit. *Supporting YTS.*
HMSO (1988). *Employment for the 1990s.* HMSO, London.
NHSTA. *Youth Training Good Practice.*
Price-Waterhouse (1987). *Feasibility Study into Youth Training Schemes in Health and Social Care Programmes.*

Further information addresses

The Training Agency,
Moorfoot,
Sheffield,
S1 4PQ.

DHSS,
Alexander Fleming House,
Elephant & Castle,
London,
SE1 6BY.

HMSO,
519 Elms Lane,
London,
SW8 5DR.

Further Education Unit
Room 5/89,
Elizabeth House,
York Road,
London,
SE1 7PH.

6

Teaching and Assessing Competence

Within the diversity of the professional Health Care Workers' role, which includes Nurses, Midwives, Health Visitors, Physiotherapists and other allied professions, there is a requirement for teaching and assessing competence in junior staff. This is not only related to those undertaking professional education courses but also the individuals in support roles such as Health Care Assistants, Auxiliaries and Care Assistants. It is a very important element of the role but one which to many staff presents problems which lead to anxiety. One of the major stumbling blocks is lack of confidence. For many professionals who are expected to undertake teaching and assessing activities, their preparation for this role is limited.

Many professionals have identified their own needs in relation to this and have undertaken courses such as City & Guilds 730 – Further Education Teacher's Certificate or courses provided by their Health Authorities, e.g. ENB 998 – Teaching and Assessing in Clinical Practice. Whichever course is undertaken the principles of teaching and assessing are the same. In order to teach, the individual needs to be able to communicate effectively at all levels.

Some people are very effective teachers without realizing their effectiveness, others know what they want their subordinates to learn and be able to do but really do not know where to start. The purpose of this section is to attempt to dispel some of the mysteries surrounding teaching which lead people to undermine their own abilities. People teach and learn as well as assess and evaluate during the course of daily living. We have all at some point been on the receiving end of a 'lecture' possibly from an irate parent – who really wanted to get a point across but wasn't

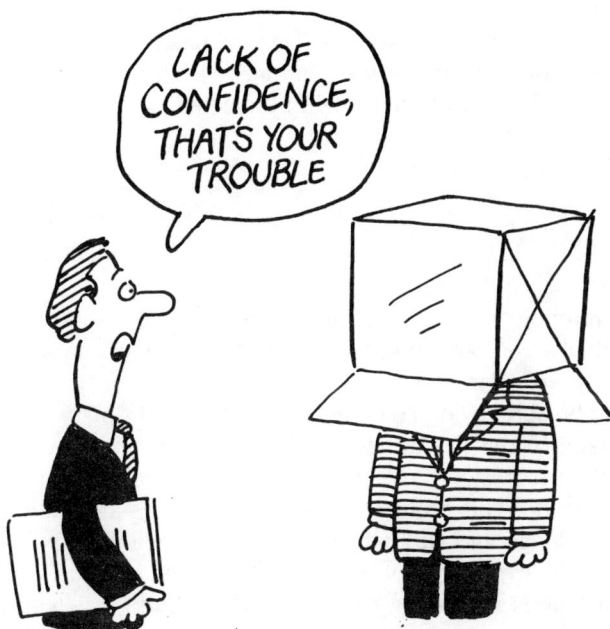

really interested in checking understanding! Or learning by experiential methods for example, touching something hot and not doing it again! There is of course the method of training we are involved in where good behaviour is rewarded. These are all ways in which we teach and learn and the basic principles apply to the teaching of individuals in the care settings. The trained nurse or other professional who works within the care settings where the skills are practised is working in an environment which is realistically the best education for learning these skills, which is in keeping with the philosophy of vocational qualifications which are based on work-orientated competency. For those who will be involved in the training programmes for Health Care Support Workers the need for preparation has been identified. The programmes of preparation will be many and varied and will be based on the local needs as identified. This information should be available from your Department of Continuing Education.

This section is not intended to prepare the reader to become a teacher but rather to offer a few tips which may help in the process. There are four basic steps to effective training:

(1) Identification of *what* has to be learned
(2) Setting the *standard* the 'learner' has to attain
(3) Decide the *aim* of the training
(4) Plan *how* the training will be carried out.

'The what'

In identifying what has to be learned an understanding of the individual's role and function is necessary. What do they need to know in order to carry out this function and what do they need to be able to do? To determine the contribution the 'learners' will make to the health care team an account must be taken of what the professional members need the supportive members to be able to do. This requires analysing the duties and determining the knowledge and skill which the 'learner' will need in order to be able to carry them out. Having decided the role the individual will play it is necessary to identify the 'Units' which make up the skill. For example if you are teaching someone to make an empty bed, what do they need to know and what do they need to be able to do? Examples of breakdowns of skill are in Chapter 7. Having decided the 'what', the standard needs to be set.

'The standard'

This relates to the level of attainment or competence and is based on the complexity of the skill being taught. For example, you would not expect someone who is new to the job to be able to perform it with the same ease as someone who is experienced. However you have set the acceptable level of performance it is important that those learning the skill have time to practice under supervision in order to become 'proficient'. Different jobs require different skills at different levels of performance and this has to be considered when training. Ask yourself if what you have set is a realistic expectation within the parameters of the role. (See Performance Criteria).

'The aim'

This is linked with the Standard in that you need to consider why the instruction is necessary and what you hope to achieve by it also what they should be able to do following the training.

'The how'

This is sorting out the way in which you are going to do the training. This includes The Sequencing – what are the essentials on which you can build? It is also determining what the individual needs to know first. The content of the training is to some extent determined by the curriculum but within this there is room for flexibility. You also need to consider the appropriate methods you could adopt for training purposes, which may include demonstration, supervised practice, and working alongside an experienced person.

Each person you will be involved with in a teaching–learning situation is a unique individual with needs specific to them. To help make their learning more effective these individual needs have to be considered. You must determine what they already know, and make the learning interesting, it is much more appropriate to involve people actively in their own learning. An important aspect of any teaching/learning situation is prompt, positive feedback.

When preparing to teach by whichever method you feel most confident in and suits the learner, a simple reminder is 'If you don't know where you are going – you won't know when you get there' which loosely translated means if you don't tell the learner what you are going to teach them and what the expected outcome is – they won't know whether they have been successful in their learning. It is important to determine in your planning what they *must* acquire in terms of skill, knowledge and attitude.

This can be embroidered by introducing skills which, if acquired, would be an added bonus but are not essential to the role, e.g. anecdotal evidence in the form of relating your experiences to emphasize a point which could add a little spice!

There are many analogies used to get this point across. One is concerning Chanel No. 5 (or perfume/after shave of your choice). If you are presented with this expensive commodity in an empty lemonade bottle – however you view it – it is still Chanel, but not very interesting. It means so much more if time is taken to wrap it up and present it in a more interesting container!

Consider the learner and what you can do to enhance their learning. People learn more effectively when:

- their contribution is perceived as valuable
- they are treated as individuals
- they feel secure and people are interested in them and their progress
- they are given appropriate feedback, i.e. praised when they do well and offered constructive comments on ways they could improve and also reassured that they are developing along the right lines
- When they know what they are supposed to be learning.

This is summarized in Fig. 6.1.

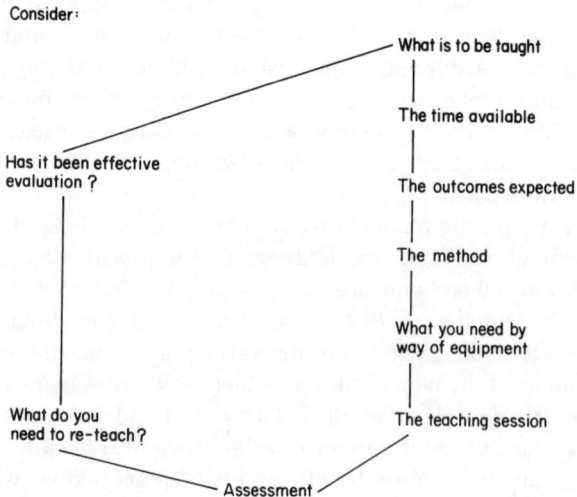

Consider:
- What is to be taught
- The time available
- Has it been effective evaluation?
- The outcomes expected
- The method
- What you need by way of equipment
- What do you need to re-teach?
- The teaching session
- Assessment

Fig. 6.1. Teaching cycle.

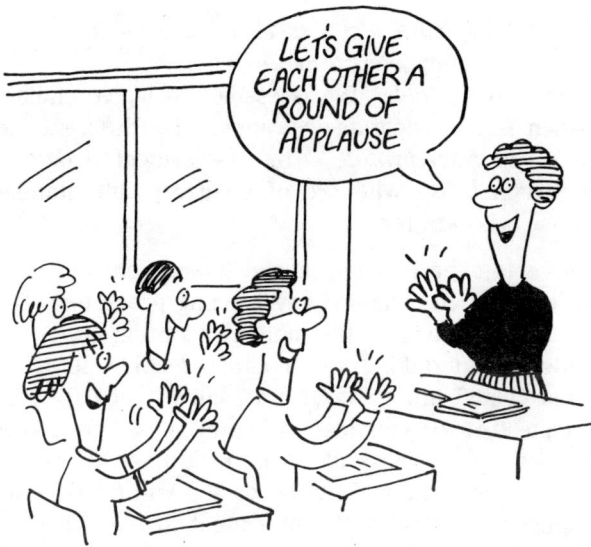

Assessment

Assessment is an integral part of the teaching and learning process. We are involved in preparing individuals to a level of competence and the purpose of assessment is to measure the skills, knowledge and attitudes which have been learned throughout a course (Scott, 1982). There are many definitions of the word 'Assessment', e.g. to judge the importance of or to evaluate (Collins English Dictionary).

The important word is 'judge' – as a person involved in the training of people undertaking courses preparing them for the role of Health Care Support Workers, you will be required to judge their competence in performing the duties assigned. Assessment in principle has a few purposes, such as helping the individual in terms of personal growth and development related to their job. It is also important as a means of the learner identifying where he or she is doing well and areas in which he or she needs to improve. An important function of assessing is to safeguard standards.

Assessment effectiveness depends on three essential factors:

(1) It must be *valid* – the assessment does in fact measure what it is supposed to measure.
(2) It must be *reliable* – the assessment will give similar results when used on separate occasions and by different assessors.
(3) It must *discriminate* – the assessment decides clearly between those who are of an acceptable standard and those who are not.

Assessment is a part of any social interaction and lies at the core of learning. In terms of any training programme it should provide a clear picture of the individual's progress.

For those undertaking the courses leading to a National Vocational Qualification (NVQ) assessment will only take place at the request of the candidate when he or she feels ready and not imposed by the curriculum or the trainer. In fairness, the candidate needs to know how he or she will be assessed. This is normally by observing the individual in naturally occurring routine work activities and judging the evidence against the performance criteria. In the selection of the evidence both the assessor and the candidate are involved to ensure equality and antidiscriminatory practice. Before the assessment takes place it has to be clear what is being assessed, and ground rules should be formulated which will probably encompass:

● When the assessment starts and finishes
● What evidence will be sought to identify competence and the methods which will be employed to gather this.

It is also important to determine how the evidence will be recorded and documented, and who will have access to this information. It is also necessary to explain how the candidate will receive the feedback on his or her performance and what arrangements will be made to resolve any problems which may arise.

Once the evidence has been gathered by the assessor it must be matched to the performance criteria and the requirements identified to determine where these have been met. Where all the elements within the unit of competence have been met and substantiated by the evidence gathered, the candidate is 'competent' in that unit. Where this is not the case and either there is insufficient evidence gathered or the candidate has not worked to an appropriate level then they are regarded as 'not yet competent' and the assessor must provide feedback to the candidate, e.g. good points, areas where improvement is required, and also how the work necessary to overcome any shortfalls will be undertaken.

How to regard the evidence gathered from the assessment again involves both assessor and candidate. The information is recorded on documents which will be provided by the Joint Awarding Bodies. Once the unit of competence has been achieved and signed by the assessor and candidate, it is placed in the candidate's national record of Vocational Achievement. When all units of competence, which are designated as an award, are complete application is made via the assessor to the Assessment Centre for the appropriate award.

Competence

Competence is a term which is often used nowadays and has a meaning and is understood by those using it, but interpretation of this varies from individual to individual. However, in an organization which is involved in ensuring the 'competence' of its workforce there needs to be a clear understanding of its meaning by all involved. There are a number of definitions of competence, see Chapter 2 for an example. Problems can arise when areas of competence are, as yet, unknown or untested. This is also true of the 'levels' of competence required and more importantly, how we know when people have reached the appropriate level to be considered competent to perform the task set. Student nurses, for example are required to demonstrate competence as set out in Rule 18 (1) – Nurses, Midwives and Health Visitors Order 1983, and this must be achieved in order to register. These competencies determine what a Registered Nurse should be able to do (see end of chapter). Similarly, people working towards an NVQ must demonstrate their competence in specified areas related to the acquisition of the NVQ. These competencies are designed to meet the needs of the employer, who is involved in both determining what is required and how

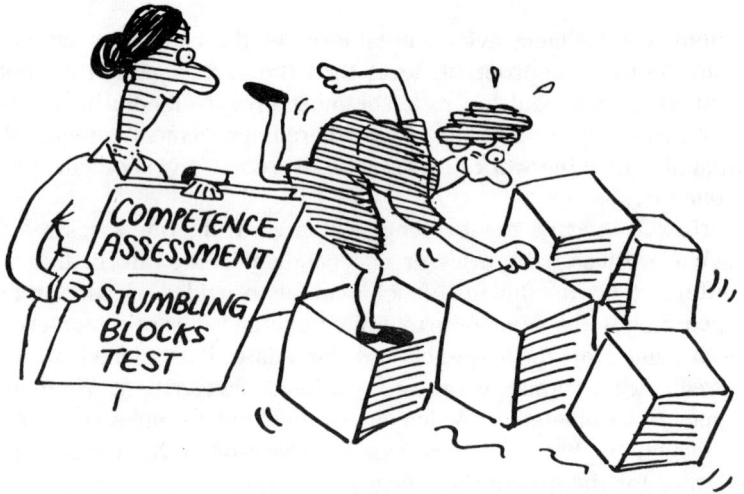

achievement is assessed. A requirement of the National Council for Vocational Qualifications (NCVQ) is that the course member's competence in the workplace is assessed by those who are working with, and supervising, them during their placements. An example is the Registered Nurse monitoring the training and development of the Health Care Assistant. Within any job which has generalist and specialist areas of work, general assumptions can be made by each area as to the competency level required of the others. Specific competence is open to speculation, which may be misdirected, but essentially there would be a certain degree of professional understanding overall.

These very general points can be translated to fit the role of the Health Care Assistant and how his or her competence may be determined. It is reasonable to assume, that for the Health Care Assistant working within the 'nursing team' or caring team the areas of competence required should not be unfamiliar to the Registered Nurse or other professionals involved in caring. For example certain clerical duties, which may be undertaken by the Health Care Assistant, are known to the professionals but are not necessarily a part of their role, and may indeed have been part of the ward clerk's duties.

Take a specific example of the Health Care Assistant working in a role to support Nurses. As indicated, the Health Care Assistant's role is to 'support' the Nurse in order to allow the Nurse to carry out nursing duties. Essentially, the related competence will be related to the role and function of the Health Care Assistant and may or may not involve the person in nursing activities – this will be determined by the Nurses. At this point it is important to mention that many of the skills in which the Health Care Assistant is required to demonstrate competence are common to all working in support roles, irrespective of the particular discipline.

Within the determined 'competencies' the NCVQ have identified different levels of achievement (see Chapter 2). Taking these into account, the job description/role specification should reflect the standards required, thus helping to prevent a situation of 'overtraining' which may prove counter-productive. By being specific in relation to the role and function of the Health Care Assistant we, as the professionals, are in an extremely powerful position of being able to create what we want from the supporters to help us do our job more effectively, and not being in the ubiquitous position of creating another level of trained Nurse. The determination of the role of the Health Care Assistant not only affects what they can and cannot do, but also what the Registered Nurses can and cannot do. The role, when determined, should not be created to provide an end in itself, but should be one which allows for individual development and progression, thereby providing a career pathway and not a dead-end job which in the future will become obsolete.

With reference to the different levels of competence, these will be determined according to the amount and type of assistance required. Some Health Authorities have instigated a programme of areas of competence required which are level related, e.g. Level I may include some portering duties or simple domestic tasks, while Level II may relate to existing Nursing Auxiliary duties.

Many Health Authorities have supported their educational establishment in developing courses to prepare Health Care Assistants. In ventures such as this the personnel involved in the implementation of the course have been party to the design of the curriculum. By doing this, the personnel who will be assessing the course members during their theoretical work and practical placements are familiar with the content of the course and the appropriate level and area of competence required. Some have used, as a basis for their course of preparation, existing courses such as BTEC or City & Guilds (see Chapter 4) which have been adapted to suit the local requirements and then validated by the appropriate Awarding Bodies.

The levels of competence can obviously be assessed once it has been determined what it is the Health Care Assistant is required to do. To help in this process the determination of 'Performance Related Criteria' is necessary (Chapter 2) with each of the competencies identified. Some of the performance-related criteria identified in relation to competence will be universal, whilst others are devised to fit in with the locally determined methods of working and individual Health Authority's policies and procedures. It is feasible to determine the role of the Health Care Assistant based on the acquisition of competence at different levels, depending on the area of work. For instance, what is seen as a requirement for demonstration appropriate to competence in Level II in one area may only be required at Level I in another. Many Nurses, and indeed other professionals, are well versed in determining strategies in the practice situation. This identification of 'what' and 'how' and the 'level' of performance required is really the same as determining 'Performance Related Criteria' although these may have been called 'objectives' instead. Those within the professional ranks who have been appointed as supervisors or assessors are familiar with this process and have probably been involved in deliberations related to the maintenance of consistency and fairness to ensure that every student is given the same opportunity and a standardized assessment. This idea, then, is not new in theory, but in practice requires those involved in the assessment of Health Care Assistants to think along slightly different lines. The following chapter will concentrate largely on the breaking down of the competencies into the various component parts; the determination of appropriate levels of competence and the strategy of assessment to ensure that the predetermined level is achieved. The examples contained are by no means meant to be definitive. They are ideas which I hope will direct your thoughts to your own ideas on what you would expect a Health Care Assistant to do in similar situations.

> Before moving on it may be relevant at this point to re-familiarize yourself with the different levels (see Chapter 2).

Information sources

Further reading

Ewan, C. and White, R. (1984). *Teaching Nursing: A Self Instructional Handbook*. Croom Helm, London.

Hinchliff, S.M. (1986). *Teaching Clinical Nursing*. Churchill Livingstone, Edinburgh.

Kershaw, B., Wright, S.G., Hammonds, P. (1989). *Helping to Care: A Handbook for Carers at Home and in Hospital*. Baillière Tindall, London.

Kenworthy, N. and Nicklin, P. (1989). *Teaching and Assessing in Nursing Practice: An Experiential Approach*. Scutari, London.

Scott, E. (1982). *The Assessment of Nurses Undertaking Post Basic Clinical Nurse Education*. JBCNS and DHSS.

7

Exploration of Competence

Having the confidence to teach is one thing! Having the confidence to judge someone else in terms of performance is another. Having the confidence to determine someone as competent is something else!

To undertake either of these requires a knowledge of what, why and how it should be done. The 'assessor' needs to be able to identify the evidence he or she requires in order to confirm someone as competent. In other words, the skill or task has been broken down into its component parts and how well the candidate is expected to perform them identified. This is the performance-related criteria.

Within the national vocational framework each of the levels has performance-related criteria (see Chapter 2). In this chapter, four areas of competence will be explored in very general terms related to Levels I, II and III.

The chosen areas of competence are applicable to any of the areas in which the Health Care Support Worker may be employed although there are probably slight variations which need to be considered in relation to the 'speciality', for example those working with children, within the mental health team, mentally handicapped adults and children, paramedical areas, and working with adults.

The areas of competence discussed are errand duties, personal hygiene, cleaning and resuscitation.

Errand duties

This element of competence forms part of the duties which may be required of the Health Care Support Worker. This may be

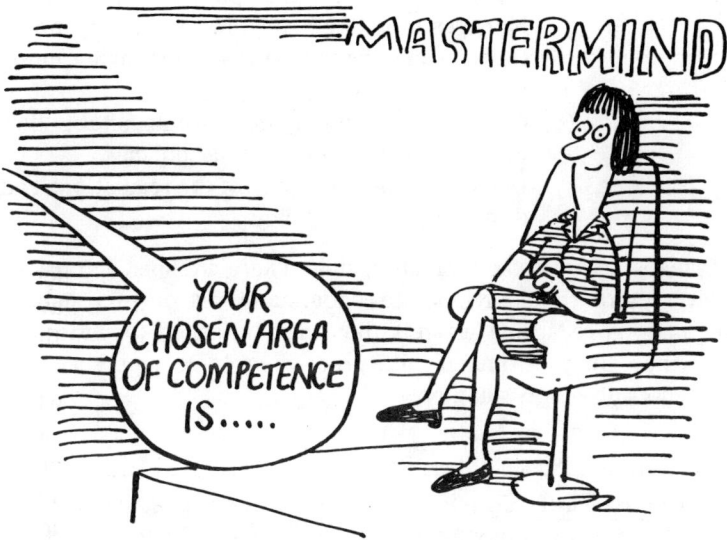

related to simple requests to take something from point A to point B. This would form a basic level of competence and performance-related criteria (listed below) which may be considered in assessing that the individual

> 'Performs errand duties conscientiously'

The *performance-related criteria* are as follows

(1) Takes note of what errand is requested
(2) Carries out duty promptly and accurately
(3) Delivers and returns any accompanying messages
(4) Complies with any appropriate hospital policy.

The overall *assessment* strategy as previously stated, specifics as follows:

Level I   – (1) Takes note of what errand is requested; performs errand exactly as requested. Notes all that is requested to do either mentally or written.

(2) Carries out duty promptly and accurately. Manages time effectively. Notes any urgencies.
(3) Delivers and returns any accompanying messages.
(4) Complies with any appropriate hospital policy. Is aware of relevant hospital policies.
Does not contravene any of the regulations laid down by hospital policy.

This is a very basic look at errands. There are specific errands that require the individual to understand reasons for certain regulations regarding errands they may be asked to undertake and these may be linked with other areas of competence, e.g. transporting blood samples.

DOWN TIME. Consider your own area of practice and the errands required of those supporting you – What other performance-related criteria would you include?

Included in this area of competence you may wish to include the involvement of the Health Care Support Worker in moving or escorting clients from one place to another, e.g. escorting a client on a journey or within the care setting from one department to another.

This is a very wide area, when considering the number of departments both within and without the health care settings which interlink to provide the service to the client. It may be that the client is being escorted to clinical appointments or social events. Whatever the reason for the client moving from one area to another there are performance-related criteria to consider which may be general or specific to the situation, e.g. the mode of transport.

It is important that the individual whose competence is being assessed has received appropriate teaching regarding the reasons for the journey, what to do in situations which may arise, and other relevant details, e.g. what to do if the client refuses to go, or who to contact at the other end to inform of the client's arrival.

Areas which you may wish to consider as a basis for determining the performance-related criteria are:

(1) How does the individual approach the client and explain the reasons?
(2) How they prepare the client prior to attending social functions.
(3) The way in which they handle the needs of the client prior to commencing.
(4) The safety of the client in transit and the arrival at the right destination at the right time.
(5) Communication skills, regarding the relaying of messages.

Obviously there would be differences in the approaches to the different client groups involved.

> **What would you determine as relevant demonstrations of competence?**

The second example above is a general area in which the appropriateness for its inclusion for the Health Care Support Worker is evident. However there may be considerable variations in approach which would be determined by the area in which the individual is working and the priorities established in relation to the care of the client. For example there would be fundamental differences between the approaches to adults and children. It may be that in the areas of mental health or people with learning difficulties the emphasis is on self help and the role of the Health Care Support Worker is as a facilitator and helper, rather than a 'doer'.

Assisting clients with personal hygiene

Assisting clients with personal hygiene:

Level I   –   Prepares facilities for a client who is largely self-caring.

Level II – Prepares facilities and assists clients who require minimal assistance.

Level III – Prepares facilities and helps the clients who cannot help themselves with hygiene needs.
This is under the direction of a qualified practitioner.

The performance related criteria for this competence at each level are as follows:

Level I – (1) Gathers and prepares equipment the client needs.
(2) Ensures a warm water supply.
(3) Ensures privacy.
(4) Accepts directions from client.

Level II – as Level I (1)–(4) plus:
(1) Assists client with difficulties, e.g. washing feet or back.
(2) Observes if client is requiring more or less assistance than on previous occasions and reports this to the qualified practitioner.

Level III – as Level I (1)–(4), plus Level II (1)–(2) plus:
(1) Gives client total assistance.
(2) Ensures patient's dignity is maintained.
(3) Practises safe lifting and moving techniques.

Overall *assessment* format as previously stated, specifics as follows:

Level I – (1) *Gathers and prepares equipment the client needs.*
Collects together all items the client is likely to need, using client's equipment where possible.
Prepares any equipment needed, i.e. washes out any bowls or baths prior to use.
Afterwards cleans and puts away, as appropriate, any equipment used.
(2) *Ensures a warm water supply.*
Ensures patient has water at a safe and comfortable temperature.
(3) *Ensures privacy.*
Draws screens, closes bathroom doors, explaining why they should be left unlocked.

(4) *Accepts directions from client.*
Respects client's wishes, within reason, as to the temperature of the water and the type of equipment needed, e.g. toothbrush.

Level II – As Level I (1)–(4) plus:

(1) *Assists client with difficulties, e.g. washing feet and back.*
Asks client if he or she requires assistance and also sees the need to offer assistance appropriately.
Does not take over from client unnecessarily.

(2) *Observes if client is requiring more or less assistance than on previous occasions and reports this to a qualified practitioner.*
Assesses patient need for assistance accurately, by observation and discussion with client.
Reports information accurately and immediately to a qualified practitioner.
Records information accurately.

Level III – As Level I (1)–(4) plus Level II (1) – (2) plus:

(1) *Gives client total assistance if necessary.*
Helps client to wash, considering amount of exposure necessary to ensure comfort.
Washes, rinses and dries adequately.
Attends to client's need to dress afterwards and undress prior to procedure.

(2) *Ensures patient's dignity is maintained.*
Shows respect for client.
Does not expose client more than is necessary.
Covers client up as quickly after washing as is reasonable.

(3) *Practises safe lifting and moving techniques.*
Does not put self, client, or colleagues in danger whilst lifting and moving the client. This applies to assistance given to get in and out of bed and in and out of bath, also to moving clients in bed if a wash is being given whilst still in bed.

Taking the identified areas in this unit of competence, there may be other criteria one would need to consider depending on the care setting in which one is involved, e.g. how different would the approach be in a residential home for the elderly or the client's own home?

For those working with babies and children what are the specifics you may need to consider in relation to preparing the equipment? Or the involvement of the parent?

In Mental Health – you may need to consider the specialist skills you may require of the Health Care Support Worker in relation to dealing with situations where clients may be confused or disorientated or potentially aggressive. What would you identify in order to make the decision regarding the individual's competence?

For those working with people with learning difficulties, the emphasis may be totally different and competence determined by the Health Care Support Worker's contribution to the 'educational process' of the individual.

There are many variations on this theme. As the professional carer one is in the situation and knows what one expects in terms of support.

Cleaning the client's environment

The following are very general examples of the competence levels required of the Health Care Support Worker. The construct is fairly open and interpretation of the competence will depend on the area of work in which the individual is involved. There may also be local differences in approach which need to be taken into consideration.

Level I – Ensures client's local environment is clean and tidy.

Level II – Ensures a clean and tidy environment recognizing that some items may need special cleaning and gaining direction from a qualified practitioner.

Level III – Ensures a clean and tidy environment, carrying out duties oneself or supervising and directing others.

The *performance-related criteria* for the competence at each level are as follows:

Level I – (1) Recognizes when environment is dirty and/or untidy.

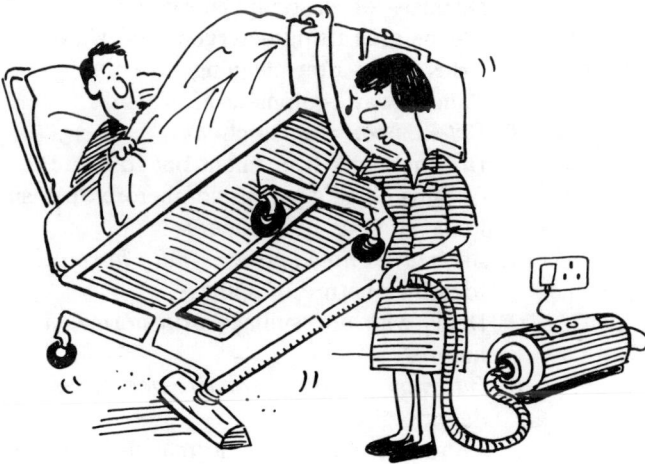

(2) Undertakes normal domestic measures to clean and tidy the environment.

(3) Extends courtesy to client.

(4) Ascertains how spillages may have occurred.

(5) Informs qualified practitioner of any 'accidents'.

Level II – As Level I (1)–(5) plus:

(1) Recognizes that normal domestic cleaning may not do for some jobs.

(2) Gets advice from qualified practitioner as to what substances to use.

Level III – As Level I (1)–(5) plus Level II (1)–(2) plus:

(1) Supervises and directs others to specific aspects.

(2) Considers Health & Safety aspects.

Overall *assessment* format as previously stated, specifics as follows:

Level I – (1) *Recognizes when environment is dirty and/or untidy.*

Observes dirty and/or untidy situations and does something about this.

(2) *Undertakes normal domestic measures to clean and tidy environment.*

Prepares equipment needed.

Disposes of waste appropriately.

Cleans area using detergent and water.

Dries areas after cleaning.

Tidies away equipment after use.

(3) *Extends courtesy to client.*

Does not talk over client but to client.

Obtains client's permission before disposing of items such as newspapers.

(4) *Ascertains how spillages may have occurred.*

Identifies nature of spillage.

Deals with any spillage of a normal domestic nature.

(5) *Informs qualified practitioner of any 'accidents'.*

Knows 'accidents' of normal domestic nature can be dealt with, but it may be important that it has happened. For example client's condition may be deteriorating in some way.

'Accidents' may be of body fluids and guidance will be needed as to how to deal with this spillage.

Level II – As Level I (1)–(5) plus:

(1) *Recognizes that normal domestic cleaning may not do for some jobs,* e.g. cleaning of certain items of equipment, which should be left for the qualified practitioner.

(2) *Gets advice from qualified practitioner as to what substances to use.*

Realizes that hospital policy may determine use of different substances in some circumstances, e.g. cleaning beds after client discharge.

Level III – As Level I (1)–(5) plus Level II (1)–(2) plus:

(1) *Supervises and directs others to specific aspect.*

Directs personnel as appropriate towards cleaning up spillages.

Supervises those who have not achieved competence in this area.

(2) *Considers Health and Safety aspects.*

Knows where a Health & Safety hazard may arise.

Informs others of possible hazards.

Obtains advice of qualified practitioner.

Emergency resuscitation procedure

Level I – Sends for appropriate assistance when a client collapses. Performs emergency resuscitation procedure.

Level II – As Level I but also hands equipment as requested to medical team.

Level III – As Level II but also anticipates need for certain equipment, and instigates emergency resuscitation procedure.

The *performance-related criteria* for this competence at each level are as follows:

Level I – (1) Recognizes that a client has collapsed (although will not differentiate between a faint or something more serious).
(2) Sends for appropriate help, i.e. qualified practitioner.
(3) Removes any object that may be blocking airway.
(4) Positions client flat on back.
(5) Tilts the bed back sufficiently to stop the tongue from falling back and blocking the airway.
(6) If in use, correctly uses an airway.
(7) Breathes into the client's mouth ensuring an adequate seal, with or without an airway, ensuring nose is blocked off.
(8) Ensures air entry by watching chest rise, allowing expiration to take place.
(9) Correctly positions hands for cardiac compression.
(10) Exerts sufficient pressure to chest to depress the chest 2.5–5.0 cm.
(11) Uses the correct rate of mouth to mouth resuscitation to external cardiac compression.
(12) Works in conjunction with another person as required and as available.

Level II – as Level I (1)–(12) plus:
(1) Hands over equipment requested to any member of resuscitation team.

Level III – as Level I (1)–(12) plus Level II (1) plus:
(1) Anticipates need for equipment required by resuscitation team.
(2) Builds on Level I competence by actually identifying that client's pulse cannot be felt.
(3) Instigates, as well as performs, emergency resuscitation procedure.

Overall *assessment* format as previously stated, specifics as follows:

Level I – (1) *Recognizes that a client has collapsed.*
Notes that client is not responding and cannot be easily roused.
Does not necessarily differentiate between a faint or a cardiac arrest.

(2) *Sends for appropriate help.*
Rings nurse call bell and asks for qualified practitioner to come to the scene.

(3) *Removes any object that may be blocking airway.*
Searches client's mouth for any obstruction whilst waiting for help.
Removes any obstruction found.
Identifies obstructions which cannot easily be removed by hand, e.g. vomit and reports to a qualified practitioner on arrival.

(4) *Positions client flat on back.*
Positions client correctly for resuscitation to take place.
Turns head to one side if full of sputum or vomit and qualified practitioner has not yet arrived.

(5) *Tilts the head back sufficiently to stop the tongue from falling back and blocking the airway.*
Performs the action once airway is determined clear.

(6) *If in use, correctly uses an airway.*
Inserts airway correctly into mouth ensuring tongue is underneath and air entry tube is directed into tongue.

(7) *Breathes into client's mouth ensuring an adequate seal with or without an airway, ensuring nose is blocked off.*
Performs mouth to mouth resuscitation in an effective manner.

(8) *Ensures air entry by watching chest rise,*

allowing expiration to take place.

Looks to see if client's chest rises.

Removes mouth from client's to allow expiration.

(9) *Correctly positions hands for cardiac compression.*

Places hands one over the other in approved manner over correct position on client's sternum.

(10) *Exerts sufficient pressure to chest to depress the chest 2.5–5.0 cm.*

Correctly positions self so as to transfer own body weight to depress client's chest.

(11) *Uses the correct rate of mouth to mouth resuscitation to external cardiac compressions.*

Knows the correct rate.

Performs the procedure at the correct rate.

(12) *Works in conjunction with another person as required and available.*

Knows how to perform as a team and how to operate in conjunction with a partner in this situation.

Level II – as Level I (1)–(12) plus:

(1) *Hands over equipment requested to any member of resuscitation team.*

Can name equipment which may need to be used.

Hands over equipment asked for, knowing which is asked for.

Level III – as Level I (1)–(12) plus Level II (1) plus:

(1) *Anticipates need for equipment required by resuscitation team.*

Anticipates what may be needed and prepares same, e.g. obtains infusion stand. This anticipation generally excludes any drugs at this level.

(2) *Builds on Level I (1) competence by actually identifying that client's pulse cannot be felt.*

Can locate client's pulse.
Can identify whether pulse is present or not.
Can therefore conclude need for emergency resuscitation.

(3) *Instigates, as well as performs, emergency resuscitation procedure.*
Having noted that emergency resuscitation is required, instigates procedure whilst ensuring that a qualified practitioner is sent for.

Example 1

Assisting clients to use toilet facilities.

Level I – Escorts clients to toilet and gives minimal assistance.

Level II – Assists clients to use toilet facilities under the direction of a qualified practitioner to determine exact client need.

Level III – Assists clients to use toilet facilities, assessing client need under the supervision of a qualified practitioner.

The *performance-related criteria* for this competence at each level are as follows:

Level I – (1) Directs client to toilet facilities.
(2) Escorts client to toilet facilities as appropriate.
(3) Ensures toilet paper is available.
(4) Ensures call bell is available before leaving.
(5) Ensures hand washing facilities are available.
(6) Assists client leaving toilet facilities as appropriate.
(7) Deals appropriately with any aids client may have throughout procedure, e.g. walking frame, wheelchair, crutches.

Level II – as Level I (1)–(7) plus:
(1) Assists client to use toilet facilities as appropriate.
(2) Assists client with cleansing, following use of toilet.

    (3) Makes relevant observations of excreta, i.e. recognizes anything not normal (not necessarily the abnormality). Measures fluid output.
Performs urinalysis and reports all findings to the qualified practitioner.

Level III – as Level I (1)–(7) plus Level II (1)–(3) plus:

    (1) Determines how client may need to travel to toilet, i.e. does client need a wheelchair?
Planned care under supervision of qualified practitioner.

    (2) Recognizes abnormalities of excreta and reports accordingly.

In order to *assess* the level, each of the performance-related criteria should be looked at in detail. How well the performance is done may affect the assessment grade if the strategy allows this.

Level I   – (1) *Directs client to toilet facilities.*
This should be assessed by observing the general approach to settle client. Essential aspects include courtesy, accuracy and appropriate method of communication, taking into account factors such as hearing and sight difficulties. How well he/she actually deals with these essentials may reflect on the grade he/she is given, if the assessment strategy allows for this. He/she should pass if the essential aspects are met. It should be noted however that a high assessment grade will not necessarily imply a higher level than the level being currently assessed.

    (2) *Escorts client to toilet facilities as appropriate.*
Recognizes if the client needs help, e.g. help to open doors, help to manoeuvre a walking frame. Recognizes if the client does not need help. Again how well this is done may affect the assessment grade.

    (3) *Ensures toilet paper is available.*
Ensures this prior to the client going to the toilet if the client would have difficulty obtaining paper once there.

(4) *Ensures call bell available before leaving.*
Sees that the call bell is within easy reach. Ensures that it is working and instructs the client properly in its use.

(5) *Ensures hand washing facilities are available.*
Ensures that there is running water, a hand cleansing solution and drying facilities.

(6) *Assists client leaving toilet facilities as appropriate.*
Returns escorted clients comfortably and safely to their base. Again appropriate communication skills should be looked for, e.g. courtesy and understanding.

(7) *Deals appropriately with any aids the client may have throughout procedure, e.g. walking frame, wheelchair, crutches.*
Removes the aids from the toilet area if there is insufficient room, ensuring that the client is safely seated on the toilet. Returns them to client immediately toileting is complete. Ensures the client's safe passage to and from the toilet.

Level II – all as above plus:

(1) *Assists client to use toilet facilities as appropriate.*
Helps client with clothing and positioning on toilet.
Helps client with cleansing after use. Ensures client is clean, dry and comfortable after use.

(2) *Assists client with cleansing following use of toilet.*
Criteria above in (1) apply, but this time the emphasis is on hand washing.

(3) *Makes relevant observations of excreta.*
Recognizes the normal excreta. Reports anything abnormal.
Accurately measures fluid output and records this.
Accurately performs urinalysis and records this. Reports all findings to the qualified practitioner in charge of the client's case.

Level III – All as for Level I and Level II plus:

    (1) *Determines how client may need to travel to toilet.*

    Ensures that the planned care determined by a qualified practitioner is carried out and that any aids required are used as necessary.

    (2) *Recognizes abnormalities of excreta and reports accordingly.*

    Describes abnormalities accurately, but need not understand the significance of the abnormality.

    Reports and records all abnormalities accurately and immediately.

    Does not give information to the client which may cause him/her to panic.

    Ensures that a qualified practitioner is aware of any of the client's fears and that they speak to them soon on the matter.

Example 2

Care of client's psychological needs.

Level I   – Listens to client's needs and gets appropriate assistance to deal with them.

Level II – Listens to client's needs and explains routine situations which may cause the client concern.

Level III – Listens to the client's needs and attends to those needs under the direction of a qualified practitioner.

The *performance-related criteria* for this competence at each level are as follows:

Level I   – (1) Adopts an open friendly manner.

    (2) Listens to client's needs.

    (3) Responds with courtesy explaining that he/she cannot deal with specific needs personally.

    (4) Enlists help from the qualified practitioner.

    (5) Does not enter into a probing or counselling situation with the client.

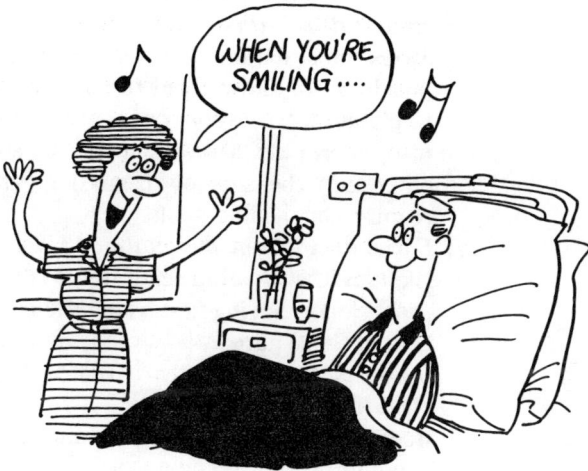

Level II   – As Level I (1)–(5) plus:
   (1) Resolves some simple fears for the client, e.g.
       describes the routines on the ward, agrees to
       pass on simple messages.
   (2) Knows when to draw the line and to stop the
       discussion.

Level III – as Level I (1)–(4) plus Level II (1)–(2) plus:
   (1) Gathers information from the client using some
       probing and counselling skills.
   (2) Knows when to call in the qualified practitioner.
   (3) Does not enter into a therapeutic relationship
       as such.

Overall *assessment* format as stated for Example 1, specifics as
follows:

Level I   – (1) *Adopts an open, friendly manner.*
                Verbal and non-verbal cues transmitted to
                others are such that this person is approachable
                and empathetic.
            (2) *Listens to client's needs.*
                Listens – does not appear disinterested, does
                not inconsiderately stop client from speaking.
                Relays accurately what the client is saying.

(3) *Responds with courtesy explaining that he/she cannot deal with specific needs personally.*

Stops the situation considerately, not abruptly, but does not allow client to go on for too long. Explains why he/she cannot enter into this discussion fully. Knows why he/she should not enter into the sort of discussion which may require counselling skills.

(4) *Enlists help from the qualified practitioner.*

Explains the situation accurately to the qualified practitioner, having first asked the client if this is what is required.

(5) *Does not enter into a probing or counselling situation with the client.*

Recognizes what a probing and counselling situation is.

Recognizes that they have not got the skills to deal with this.

Explains this properly and empathetically to the client.

Enlists appropriate help.

Level II – as Level I (1)–(5) plus:

(1) *Resolves some simple fears for the client,* e.g. describes routines on the ward, agrees to pass on simple messages.

Knows what is reasonable to attend to.

Attends to minor worries caused by hospitalization. Passes on simple messages to appropriate people.

(2) *Knows when to draw the line and stop the discussion.*

Knows what is unreasonable to attend to. Explains empathetically to client why cannot attend to it. Enlists help of qualified practitioner. When nature of problem determined, explains to client next course of action, gains client agreement, calls for qualified practitioner.

(3) *Does not enter into a therapeutic relationship as such.*

Knows what is meant by a therapeutic relationship. Does not lead the client into thinking it is what may develop.

Example 3

| Assisting clients to mobilize. |

Level I – Ensures that there is no hindrance to client's self mobility.

Level II – Assists client to mobilize using a variety of aids as prescribed by the qualified practitioner.

Level III – Decides how best client may be encouraged to mobilize in conjunction with the qualified practitioner.

The *performance-related criteria* for this competence at each level are as follows:

Level I   – (1) Ensures that floor areas are free from spillages.
        (2) Ensures adequate passage between furniture.
        (3) Ensures furniture is positioned so as not to cause a hazard.

Level II – as Level I (1)–(3) plus:
        (1) Identifies a qualified practitioner.
        (2) Ensures equipment suitable for use.
        (3) Communicates adequately with client.
        (4) Makes appropriate records of events.

Level III – as Level I (1)–(3) plus Level II (1)–(4) plus:
        (1) Supervises others enabling clients to mobilize.
        (2) Ensures client's care plan is adhered to by those they are supervising.
        (3) Discusses client progress with qualified practitioner to decide how client may best proceed.

Overall *assessment* format as previously stated, specifics as follows:

Level I   – (1) *Ensures that floor areas are free from spillages.*
        (2) *Ensures adequate passage between furniture to allow for mobilization,* e.g. the need for enough room for those using walking frames, etc.

(3) *Ensures furniture positioned so as not to cause a hazard.*

Ensures adequate passage as in (2).

Ensures furniture which may be used as an aid is safe, e.g. all beds should have brakes on when stationary.

Level II – as Level I (1)–(3) plus:

(1) *Correctly identifies aid for mobilization as prescribed by qualified practitioner.*

Gives client encouragement and support to use aid.

Gives client instruction as to use of aid as appropriate.

Ensures prescribed aid is the one chosen for use.

Knows why the particular aid may be the most appropriate.

(2) *Ensures equipment suitable for use.*

Ensures equipment in good working order.

Ensures equipment clean before and after use.

(3) *Communicates adequately with client.*

Ensures eye to eye contact.

Ensures appropriate use of touch to help client.

Listens to client's fears or apprehension regarding use of equipment.

Reports on resolved fears to qualified practitioner.

(4) *Makes appropriate records of events.*

Notes client's progress and reports to qualified practitioner in verbal and written form.

Level III – as Level I (1)–(3) plus Level II (1)–(4) plus:

(1) *Supervises others enabling clients to mobilize.*

Ensures enabler has all information necessary to assist client.

Observes that enabler performs task correctly.

(2) *Ensures client's care plan is adhered to by those they are supervising.*

Points out relevant details on care plan and observes as stated above in (1).

(3) *Discusses client's progress with qualified prac-*

titioner to decide how client may best proceed.
Evaluates use of aid prescribed for client under
direction of qualified practitioner.
Suggests change of equipment to suit client's
needs.

Example 4

> Assisting clients with eating and drinking.

Level I – Prepares relatively self-caring clients for eating
and drinking.
Level II – as Level I but also assists clients who cannot
manage themselves, but who can swallow
adequately, to eat and drink.
Level III – as Level II, but can also suggest suitable nutritional
intake in consultation with qualified practitioner.

The *performance-related criteria* for the competence at each
level are as follows:

Level I – (1) Assists client to dining area as appropriate.
(2) Enables the client to find a comfortable position.
(3) Ensures client's hygiene and toileting needs are
met in relation to enjoying a meal.
(4) Ensures dentures, if used, are in place.
(5) Ensures client's clothing is protected as necessary.
Level II – as Level I (1)–(3) plus:
(1) Promotes suitable environment for eating and
drinking.
(2) Ensures client has adequate and appropriate
utensils for eating and drinking.
(3) Ensures food is at correct temperature.
(4) Assists client to eat and drink at a comfortable
rate.
(5) Encourages self sufficiency in client.
(6) Reports and records any difficulties.
Level III – as Level I (1)–(5) plus Level II (1)–(6) plus:
(1) Supplementary foods are suggested and given

in consultation with qualified practitioner.

(2) Client's food and drink intake is monitored.

(3) Any adverse reactions to food or drink are reported.

Overall *assessment* format as previously stated, specifics as follows:

Level I – (1) *Assists client to dining area as appropriate.*
Helps client who needs minimal assistance to arrive at dining area.
Gains client's permission for the duty. Is courteous towards client.

(2) *Enables the client to find a comfortable position.*
Helps client to find a seat both physically and psychologically suitable.

(3) *Ensures client's hygiene and toileting needs are met in relation to enjoying a meal.*
Escorts client to toilet and enables hand to be washed as necessary.
Also enables teeth to be cleaned as necessary.
Ensures same facility after meal.

(4) *Ensures dentures, if worn, are in place.*
Ensures client's dentures are available and assistance given with fitting and cleaning as necessary.

(5) *Ensures client's clothing is protected as necessary.*
Offers use of napkins, etc. for client's use.

Level II – as Level I (1)–(5) plus:

(1) *Promotes suitable environment for eating and drinking.*
Helps to create pleasant, quiet and sociable atmosphere in clinical area, at all times, but especially in this instance, at mealtimes.
Ensures eating area is clean and tidy.

(2) *Ensures client has appropriate and adequate utensils for eating and drinking.*
Ensures special aids are available, clean and

ready for use.

Instructs client as to correct use of aids.

(3) *Ensures food is at correct temperature.*

Food should be neither too hot nor too cold and as such should be appetizing in this context.

Contingency measures should be made if food is too hot or too cold.

(4) *Assists client to eat and drink at a rate comfortable to them.*

Food should be offered at a rate and in an amount comfortable to the client.

Food should be presented in an appetizing way and should not appear over-facing, nor should there be too little.

(5) *Encourages self sufficiency in client.*

Has patience to allow clients to do things for themselves.

Does not expect too much of client, however.

(6) *Reports and records any difficulties.*

Notes and reports any difficulties the client may have to the qualified practitioner.

Level III – as Level I (1)–(5) plus Level II (1)–(6) plus:

(1) *Supplementary foods are suggested and given in consultation with qualified practitioner.*

Assesses and monitors client's intake.

Suggests appropriate supplements.

Knows overall nutritional value of common supplements, e.g. Complan.

(2) *Client's food and drink intake is monitored.*

Makes accurate records of client's intake.

Reports facts to qualified practitioner.

(3) *Reports any adverse reactions to food or drink.*

Recognizes and reports adverse reactions to food or drink, e.g. difficulties in chewing or swallowing.

Consults with qualified practitioner.

Information sources

Robinson, J., Stillwell, J., Hawley, C. and Hempstead, N. (1989). *The Role of the Support Workers in the Ward Health Care Team.* Nursing Policy Study No. 6 N.P.S. Centre & Health Services Research Unit. University of Warwick.

SCOTVEC. *The Support Worker in the Scottish Health Service.* RCN Scottish Board.

8

The National Standards of Competence

The production of this document is mentioned in Chapter 3. Having read through the preceding chapter exploring competence you may now wish to consider how to determine the level of competence of those working in support roles. This chapter is designed to give you a brief but hopefully enlightening overview of the National Standards of competence. Using this chapter and the preceding chapter may help to clarify your own particular needs in relation to training and assessment strategies at local level.

The National Standards document is substantial and identifies the performance-related criteria in relation to the units and elements of competence and is essential for those involved in training of Health Care Support Workers in any area. The document was issued in April 1990 and identifies the contribution to care appropriate to those in support roles.

The 'Standards' identify a number of key roles for the Health Care Support Worker in relation to:

(1) Their contribution to the quality of care.
(2) The support required to the professions and in specific programmes of therapy and treatment.
(3) The provision of assistance to clients.
(4) Their role in supporting the client in developing skills in relation to daily living.
(5) Their role related to maintaining the environment in which the care is set.

Within each of the identified key roles there are identified *units of competence* which are subdivided into the *elements of competence* (see Chapter 2).

Example

Having identified a *key role* in relation to the Health Care Support Worker's contribution to the *quality of care* there have been areas determined in which the Care Worker needs to demonstrate skill and knowledge in order to be seen as competent. These include promoting and supporting the client's rights which can be further broken down into specific elements such as:

(1) Assisting the client to exercise his or her rights.
(2) Freedom of choice and supporting the client in terms of personal worth and helping the client to practise his or her beliefs.

The evidence the assessor will require in order to assess the individual's level of competence is related to the determined performance criteria for each of the above elements. If successful, the candidate is then competent in the 'unit', i.e. related to quality (see Chapter 2).

The standards have been submitted to the National Council for Vocational Qualifications (NCVQ) by the Joint Awarding Bodies for accreditation as National Vocational Qualification (NVQ). With these standards identified, both Level I and Level II qualifications are included. Some of the standards are within the Levels I and II, others are set at either Level I or Level II.

The units of competence related to 'direct personal care' include aspects of the Support Worker's role in his/her contribution to:

(1) Comfort.
(2) Care of a deceased person.
(3) Support (the client and professional worker during clinical treatment and investigation).
(4) Assisting with nutritional intake.

These are set at NVQ Level I.

The units of competence related to 'enablement care' include the Care Worker's contribution to:

(1) Supporting the client and professional during activity programmes.
(2) Supporting carers and clients in a home environment.

These are set at NVQ Level II.

The remaining units include:

(1) Supporting client's rights.
(2) Assisting client regarding participation in recreational activities.
(3) Maintaining personal hygiene.
(4) Mobility.
(5) Assisting client meet his/her nutritional needs.

These are common to both Level I and Level II qualifications.

The examples included are not exhaustive but are an indication of how the document is formulated. Each of the elements of competence contained within the National Standards document is shown as part of the appropriate unit of competence. Also included on each page is a statement regarding the situations in which the individual must be competent plus information related to the evidence required. This encompasses the 'performance evidence' which carries the greatest weighting and is supported by the 'knowledge' weighting.

The following is an interpretation of information contained in the National Standards document.

Under the key role of contribution to the quality of care, one of the elements identified as a requirement for competence on the part of the Health Care Support Worker is in relation to those 'clients who exhibit challenging behaviour'. The unit used to describe the guidance given to all concerned in the acquisition and determining of competence is management of violent or destructive behaviour.

The performance-related criteria cover the summarizing of the Care Worker's actions in terms of self protection and minimizing risks to the client, self and others. Also taken into account are the prevailing circumstances and aftermath in relation to injuries which may have been sustained or the feelings of the individual following the incident.

The evidence required to assess the competence of the individual in this situation is divided into performance and knowledge requirements.

Performance evidence requires the individual to demonstrate over a period of time, sufficient evidence of competence in relation to the specified *range* of activities which includes working within a specific setting, either hospital, residential, or day-care establishments, with any individual client who may exhibit aggressive, violent or destructive behaviour. It includes dealing with attacks directed at others or self abuse with or without the use of weapons. It also requires the individual to demonstrate an understanding of the basic principles associated with self protection with reference to legal requirements and the organization's policy regarding untoward occurrences in relation to seclusion or restraint (physical, mechanical, or chemical). Observation of the interaction between the Care Worker and others including relatives, team members, etc. is involved.

The second evidence requirement is related to *knowledge* and explores issues such as record keeping, what can be done to prevent violent or aggressive outbursts, and explanation of the individual's own reactions to the situation in which they were involved.

The performance and knowledge evidence collectively give the assessor and the candidate a comprehensive picture of what competence in this unit entails. Full details can be obtained from the NHSTA address included in Chapter 3.

Information sources

NHSTA. *National Occupational Standards.*

9

Where to Next?

Some of the questions posed by people entering a course of training to prepare them for a support role within the health care team will probably relate to opportunities available to them in terms of progression. Or they may assume that having undertaken the initial course there is not much else available if they wish to remain within the role of Health Care Assistant. This chapter will explore some of the opportunities available to those who:

(1) Wish to continue studies in order to gain entry to professional education.
(2) Wish to remain in a supportive role but want to undertake 'other courses'.
(3) Wish to remain in the supportive role but develop their clinical skills.
(4) Wish to remain in a health care role but not necessarily hospital/nursing orientated.

This chapter will also consider possible routes available for those people working as Auxiliary Nurses who may want to progress. It is important that in considering Health Care Assistant roles within the team that experienced Auxiliaries are not disadvantaged and opportunities that take into account their experience and prior learning are available to them.

The Health Care Assistant, having undertaken the initial course leading to a vocational qualification awarded by one of the validating bodies, can use this qualification as a foundation on which to build other units leading towards a qualification acceptable to the United Kingdom Central Council for Nursing, Midwifery and Health Visiting (UKCC) as entry to professional education. An example of how this would work follows.

After completion of the course leading to the award of a

Business and Technical Education Council (BTEC) First Certificate in Caring, the Health Care Assistant could undertake additional units and obtain a BTEC First Diploma which enables them to undertake a BTEC National Diploma course over a period of time (see Chapter 4). Having been successful in the BTEC National Diploma, which is an acceptable entry qualification recognized by the UKCC, the individual is then eligible to apply for professional education. This does not guarantee acceptance to a course of study but does open up the opportunity for consideration through the same channels as everyone else wishing to enter this type of educational programme (Fig. 9.1).

For many Auxiliaries already in post, courses of instruction will have been provided by their Health Authorities. In some instances these will have included a detailed programme of instruction whilst others adopt an *ad hoc* basis with the in-service training department responding to identified needs, and then providing relevant courses. It is unlikely that any member of the Auxiliary workforce has not been given any instruction at all. As with all members of the health care team, the Auxiliary and indeed the Health Care Assistant have a very important role

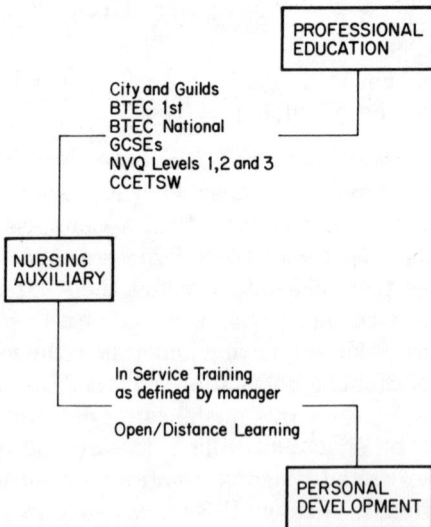

Fig. 9.1. The way forward for Nursing Auxiliaries.

to fulfil which merits recognition. Auxiliary is defined as a person that gives help, and Care Assistant as someone who helps or assists.

In essence the Auxiliary or Care Assistant works as part of a team in order to help the qualified members fulfil their roles more effectively. Recognizing the contribution made by Care Assistants/Auxiliaries incorporates those areas related to opportunities for progression and also takes into account their previous learning and practical ability. Taking cognizance of this fact it is important that a system of accrediting this previous learning towards exemptions exists on the course of training for Health Care Assistants. Failure to award 'points' towards the course based on prior learning/experience is devaluing the contribution they have made and may be perceived by the person concerned, as their knowledge and experience being of little importance and counting for nothing.

With this in mind, colleges providing courses of training for Health Care Assistants are developing or have developed a system of Accreditation of Prior Learning (APL) (see Chapter 2). For example, an Auxiliary wishing to undertake the course may be exempt from undertaking a particular module since he or she has already completed a similar course as part of an in-service training programme and is not required then to do the 'whole' course but is 'slotted in' appropriately. Instead of taking the 12 months to complete the course, he/she may be able to accrue enough credits in 9 months. Many people working within this type of role are undertaking a number of courses, provided by either their Health Authority or local flexible learning centres, which can be credited towards a recognizable qualification such as BTEC (see Chapter 4). These could be credited towards the course of preparation for Health Care Assistants for both the Nursing Auxiliary or the equivalent in social services, and the Health Care Assistant. There are a number of such provisions made by Local Colleges of Further Education in the courses offered.

Colleges of Further Education offer individuals a variety of courses in a wide range of study modes and provide the opportunity to climb the ladder of success in order to enter professional career structures, up-date existing skills, or even to re-think career pathways and change course if so desired. In keeping with current demands, Colleges are continually adapting to change in order to meet the specific needs of the user. The demographic trends predicted to affect the nursing profession over the next 5 years are now being experienced by the Colleges of Further Education. It would be impossible to do justice to the range and diversity of the courses offered by the Colleges in this short account of what may be available in terms of appropriate courses for Health Care Assistants. The intention therefore is to give some examples of the routes which may be appropriate for career advancement and also give some direction to those involved in the training of the student in the workplace.

Access courses

A proportion of the people entering the Health Care Assistant programme and other programmes designed for those working in a support role may wish to continue with their studies in order to enter professional education. An access course provides an alternative route and does not necessarily involve the acquisition of traditional qualifications such as GCSEs or 'A' levels. It is important to note that, in order for an access course to be acceptable as an entry route to Nurse Education, it has to be approved by the UKCC. Although these courses are aimed primarily at the adult population, the mature student, this does not preclude young adults from commencing a course of this nature. Entry to this type of course takes into account the learning experiences of the individual together with prior achievement. Access courses were developed, as the name would suggest, to create opportunities for those who could not overcome the barriers which inhibited them from re-entering education, e.g. individuals who were limited because of family commitments or in receipt of certain benefits, which if they entered full-time education courses, they might lose. The access course is flexible enough to meet the needs of individuals in an attempt to rectify the situation whereby opportunities were denied because of circumstances. This type of course may not be appropriate for some people who may opt for a different mode of study, e.g. open or distance learning.

Distance learning

This form of study does not involve face-to-face contact between the student and the tutor or, if it is offered, it is very limited. Many of the open and distance learning packages offered by the Colleges of Further Education have been validated by one of the examining bodies and carry credits which could be accrued towards the award of a vocational qualification. Because of the flexibility of structure of modules on open and distance learning courses many students take advantage of being able to study at a time that is convenient to them and which fits in with their life pattern.

On a number of the training courses for Health Care Workers the successful completion results in the award of a BTEC First Certificate in Caring Skills. Opportunities are available within the Colleges of Further Education for people with the First Certificate to continue their study along the BTEC pathway as described earlier in this chapter. Similarly the City and Guilds of London Institute offers those undertaking courses designed by them to continue their study with Colleges on a part-time basis.

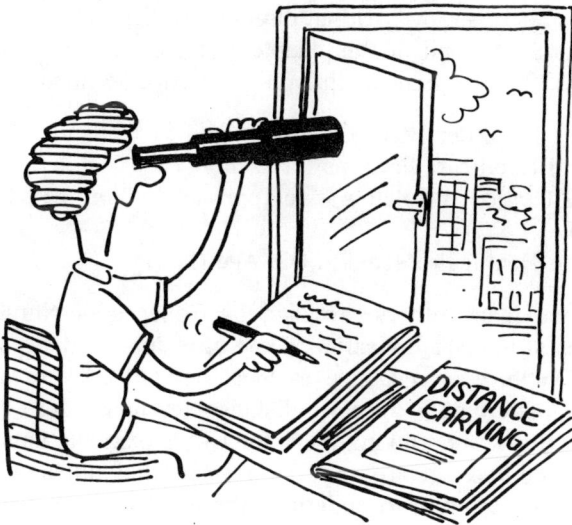

Flexistudy

Colleges of Further Education also offer the more traditional qualifications such as GCSEs and 'A' levels. In order to attract a wider user group they are often offered on a flexistudy system, in which the student is linked with a named tutor at the College, who acts as mentor and guide to the student during the course. Because it is a flexi system the student can determine when and where study takes place. However, a requirement is that the student and tutor meet on a regular basis to discuss problems and progress, thus allowing the student to gain maximal benefit from the course.

The types of courses vary considerably. The opportunities for people to undertake courses are equally as varied and may include evening classes at local Colleges or distance learning via the Open University, or a combination of both. Many Colleges and flexible learning centres provide afternoon and evening classes for those involved in caring. The courses may be specific courses outlined by the Open University. These are very attractive courses in that the content is relevant and the mode of study flexible with the advantage of carrying a credit rating. Information can be obtained by writing directly to the Open University (address at the end of this chapter) or by contacting the local Colleges. Popular titles in this range of courses include:

Caring for Older People (P650)
Mental Handicap: Patterns for Living (P555)
Rehabilitation: A Collaborative Approach to Work with Disabled People (P556)
Mental Health Problems in Old Age (P557).

There are many others provided by Colleges of Nursing and Colleges of Further Education, some of which are undertaken as a joint venture in response to local demands. There are also available alternative open or distance learning courses which prepare those undertaking them for GCSE examinations or self learning courses in areas of interest to the individual. Many Auxiliaries may wish to undertake these flexistudy courses as a means of obtaining a qualification which is nationally recognized and/or meets the requirement for entry to professional Nurse Education. Others may want to undertake this type of course as a means of improving their understanding of the complexities of health care in various settings in order to provide a more efficient and effective contribution to the caring team, without a wish to change their role.

For those who have experience working within the caring team and wish to remain in a care role but not necessarily related to 'Nursing', some courses may be available at the local College, e.g. courses for Chiropody Assistants, Child Minders or Play Therapists. It may be that having undertaken the course the person wishes to 'specialize' in a particular aspect of care, e.g. working with children. Many local Colleges offer courses which enable the individual to acquire relevant knowledge and skills, e.g. a Nursery Nursing course.

The National Nursery Examination Board

A number of individuals undertaking courses for the preparation of the Health Care Assistant may express an interest in working with children. This may be a result of their experience in the paediatric areas or the reason they wanted to undertake the course in the first place. It may be, having completed the course, that they want to become more experienced or to gain a recognized qualification in relation to working with children, but not wish to undergo nurse training. In this situation there is an avenue open to them. Many Colleges of Further Education throughout the United Kingdom offer courses leading to the qualification validated by the National Nursery Examination Board (NNEB).

These courses provide education and training for those who wish to gain employment as qualified nursery nurses in a variety of settings. This course prepares the student in terms of the knowledge, skills and competence required of the nursery nurse and also encourages personal and professional development. Courses are normally undertaken on a full-time basis over 2 years, but many colleges are now approved to run non-standard courses on a part-time basis over a longer period, usually 3 years.

The NNEB does not require formal qualifications for entry to this course, but the prospective student must be at least 16 years old.

The course

The course duration extends to 350 days of full-time study and an appropriate number of days part time. These days consist of both theory and practical application of theory in work placements. There are seven principal subject areas contained within the framework of the course:

(1) Children's growth and development.
(2) Physical development and keeping children healthy.
(3) Cognitive development and learning through play.
(4) Emotional development.
(5) Social relationships.
(6) The rights and responsibilities of children and the family.
(7) The nursery nurse in employment.

The above coursework relates to children between the age range 0–7 years old.

The practical placements form an integral part of the course and afford the student the opportunity to apply the theoretical knowledge to the practical situation, at the same time working alongside experienced professionals from whom they can learn the *how* of being a competent carer and determine their own developmental needs in terms of the course.

The qualification is awarded to those students who complete the course successfully by passing the three elements required, which are:

(1) A pass in their coursework.
(2) A pass in their practical placements.
(3) A pass in the final examination which comprises
    (a) a Multiple Choice Question Paper (MCQ)
    (b) an essay paper.

The employment opportunities for successful students vary both in the United Kingdom and abroad. However, the demand for qualified Nursery Nurses is high, and most successful students find little difficulty in finding a job.

The qualification equips the Nursery Nurse to work in a variety of settings which include working within the Health Care Sector in hospitals, or within Social Services working in day nurseries. Within the Private Sector there are also numerous opportunities for the qualified Nursery Nurse to work as Nannies. Within the Education Sector many Nursery Nurses are employed in primary schools or work with children with special educational needs. Some may decide to embark on a self-employment role and register with the Local Authorities as Child Minders.

Once qualified, the Nursery Nurse has the opportunity to undertake post qualifying courses provided by the NNEB in order to undertake advanced study in a specialist area, or they may decide that they wish to proceed to professional Nurse Education.

Social Work

The other major caring profession is Social Work and this may be the area of care in which the individual wishes to develop. Qualifications for Social Workers can be obtained through diploma or degree studies or, in some instances, special schemes, which may be of particular interest to mature entrants. These are designed for people who have no formal qualifications but have experience, aptitude and motivation to undertake them.

They may accredit qualifications obtained as a result of a Health Care Assistant course or other courses in care, e.g. Preliminary Certificate in Social Care. Many centres are particularly interested in the older person who has family commitments, and, as with other courses, e.g. the access courses to nursing, financial aid is available (see end of chapter for address regarding more information). A number of entrants to this type of course may wish to enter professional education leading to the Certificate of Qualification in Social Work (CQSW). This is the recognized qualification for Social Workers and is approved by the Central Council for Education and Training in Social Work (CCETSW).

Providing the individual can meet the entry criteria set by CCETSW he or she may secure a place on a course leading to qualification in Social Work. There are different courses available, details of which can be obtained from the Social Work Advisory

Service (SWAS). Entrance to the course leading to CQSW is offered to suit people with different academic backgrounds.

There is a 4-year degree course for people leaving school with University entrance qualifications. This incorporates professional Social Work training into the degree programme. For individuals who have relevant degrees or diplomas there is a 1-year post-graduate course, and for graduates with degrees in 'non relevant' subjects, a 2-year post graduate course. Some of these courses offered in Universities and Polytechnics can lead to higher degrees.

In some Universities and Polytechnics courses for non-graduates are available. To be eligible to enter this type of course, the prospective student must be at least 20 years of age. If under the age of 25 years the candidate must have a minimum of five GCSEs or two 'A' levels or the equivalent. If the candidate is over 25 years, he or she may be considered without these qualifications providing the candidate can prove his/her ability to study at an advanced level. Universities and Polytechnics may require the prospective student to undertake an entrance test.

In some instances the Health Care Assistant or Auxiliary may, because of the time involved, not wish to embark on this route of development but is highly motivated to enter professional education. Without the statutory requirements in terms of qualifications this portal was not open. However, there is available a 'test' which, if undertaken successfully opens up an opportunity for the individual to apply to enter nursing as a student. This is the 'DC Test' (Fig. 9.2).

The DC Test

Another way in which a person may gain entry to a pre-registration course is to complete successfully an entrance test approved by the UKCC. This test is known as the DC Test, and the achievement of a pass mark affords those people who do not have the relevant required statutory entry qualifications the opportunity to apply for a pre-registration course leading to registration in any of the following parts of the Professional Register:

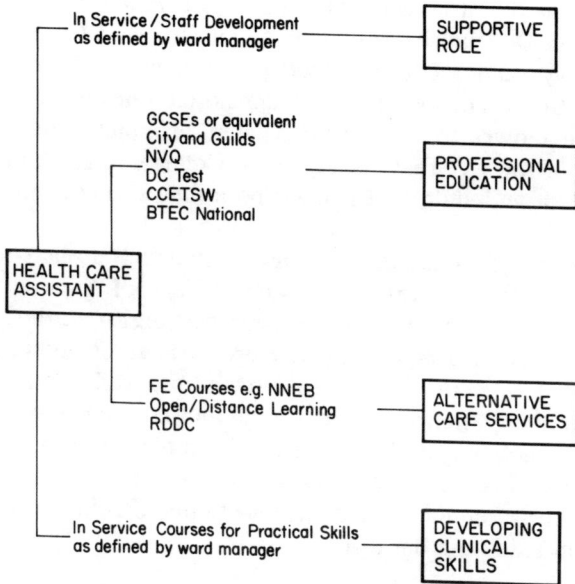

Fig. 9.2. The way forward for Health Care Support Workers.

Part 1 – Registered General Nurse (RGN)
Part 3 – Registered Mental Nurse (RMN)
Part 5 – Registered Nurse for Mental Health (RNMH)
Part 8 – Registered Sick Children's Nurse (RSCN)
Part 12 – Adult Nursing
Part 13 – Mental Health Nursing
Part 14 – Mental Handicap Nursing
Part 15 – Nursing the Child

The test was designed to measure the candidate's ability to cope with the demands of Nurse Education. There are three different tests which are the same in terms of degree of difficulty and format. Success in the test means the person is eligible to apply through the Nurses' and Midwives' Central Clearing House (NMCCH), it does not mean a place on a pre-registration course will be offered automatically.

The three tests are known as DC1, DC2 and DC3. Those undertaking the test are allowed only *one* attempt at each test.

If, for example, the candidate does not reach the required standard in DC2 he/she is eligible to sit DC1 or DC3 providing that 14 days at least have lapsed between sitting DC2 and an attempt at either of the others. Under no circumstances will the person be allowed to 're-sit' DC2. The cut-off point at pass mark for each of the DC Tests is 51 (some Colleges may stipulate a higher mark and state that it must be a first sitting of the test) and above.

Not all Colleges offer the test and those which do may not be offering the test as entrance to their College of Nursing. Most Colleges make a small charge to those wishing to sit the test.

The DC Test is designed to measure a range of abilities and is divided into sections. The areas tested are verbal reasoning, numerical ability, non-verbal reasoning and comprehension. The first three sections of the test have example questions which give the candidate the opportunity to practice. The test takes about 1 hour to complete and each section is carefully timed by the person assessing the test.

Sections of the DC Test

Section 1 – Verbal Reasoning

This section tests the candidate's ability to understand and use the ideas which are expressed in either numbers, words, letters or combinations of both.

Section 2 – Numerical Ability

This section tests the candidate's arithmetical skills and incorporates conversion of fractions to decimal, addition, subtraction, multiplication and division. It also includes graphs and charts from which the candidates determine their answers.

Section 3 – Non-verbal Reasoning

This section deals with the candidate's ability to solve perceptual and special problems.

Section 4 – Comprehension

This is the only section which does not carry test/practice questions. A series of English passages are given and the candidate is required to answer questions based on them.

The DC Test is administered by each College of Nursing in *exactly* the same way. The person conducting the test has a series of instructions to follow, thus providing uniformity.

For many people, the test itself is a nerve-racking experience. To help those who wish to undertake the DC Test but who have not been involved in study for some time, or for those who just want to know more about it, there is a book available giving further information (see end of chapter for address). The book contains examples of the type of questions involved.

Each section contains questions ranging in degree of difficulty and each section is timed. It is important that candidates undertaking the test work quickly and accurately. As stated earlier, the Colleges of Nursing administering the test all do so in the same way. However the frequency and post-test administration may vary, e.g. when results are available, and when the candidate is notified.

These various courses are some of the possible ways the Care Assistant or Auxiliary can progress toward professional education. Having gained an NVQ or other qualification acceptable for entry to Nursing Education or achieved a 'Pass' in the DC Test, the individual is now in possession of a 'qualification' which opens the door to application. In the past, individuals applied directly to the hospital of their choice but this system no longer applies. Applications for entry to Nurse Education have been centralized for processing and anyone wishing to apply must obtain the relevant forms from the NMCCH.

NMCCH (Nurses' and Midwives' Central Clearing House)

The 'Clearing House' is a department of the English National Board for Nursing, Midwifery and Health Visiting (ENB) and its function is to centralize the application process system. This is for full-length pre-registration courses in Nursing and Midwifery in England, and also the Post Qualification course for Registered Sick Children's Nurse (RSCN). It does not deal with applications for:

- degrees in nursing
- conversion courses
- post basic clinic courses
- post registration courses (except RSCN)
- any courses offered in educational establishments and training institutions outside England.

The courses available through the NCCH system are as follows:

First Level Courses:
Registered General Nurse (RGN)
Registered Mental Nurse (RMN)
Registered Nurse for the Mentally Handicapped (RNMH)
Registered Sick Children's Nurse (RSCN)

Project 2000 Courses:
Adult Nursing
Mental Health Nursing
Mental Handicap Nursing
Nursing the Child

Applications to the NMCCH for any of the mentioned courses can be made up to 2 years in advance providing the applicant is at least 16 years of age, and can meet the statutory entry requirements.

These entry requirements are set by law and are the *minimum* acceptable for entry to professional Nurse Education. Individual Colleges of Nursing and Midwifery may set their own entry criteria providing they are not below the standard required by law, e.g. a College may require passes in specific subjects such as English Language or a Science subject. This needs to be considered before applications are submitted. It is also important to note that the statutory entry requirements for Nursing and Midwifery are different. Full details of entry requirements are contained in the Applicant's Handbook from the NCCH.

Pre-registration first level nursing courses

Briefly, the entrance requirements are:

(1) A minimum of 5 GCSEs or 'O' level grade 'C' or above.
(2) A minimum of 5 subjects at standard grade (1, 2 or 3) or Ordinary Grade (A, B or C) in Scottish Certificate of Education.
(3) A minimum of 5 GCSEs.

The minimum statutory requirements for entry to a Nurse preparation course leading to qualification to parts 1, 3, 5, 8, 12, 13, 14 or 15 of the register are specified in Rule 16 (1) (a)–(f) of the Nurses, Midwives and Health Visitor (Registered Fever Nurses Amendment Rules and Training Amendment Rules) Approval order 1989 (No. 1456). These are either:

(1) A minimum of five subjects any of which may be obtained in the General Certificate of Secondary Education in England and Wales grade A, B or C, or at Ordinary level grade A, B or C in the General Certificate of Education of England and Wales or at Grade 1 in the Certificate of Secondary Education, or
(2) A minimum of the subjects any of which may be obtained at Ordinary or Standard Grade, grade 1, 2 or 3, or at Ordinary Grade (bands A, B or C) in the Scottish Certificate of Education, or
(3) A minimum of five subjects any of which may be obtained in the General Certificate of Secondary Education in Northern Ireland, grade A, B or C, or at grade A, B or C in the Northern Ireland General Certificate of Education at Ordinary level, or passes in the examination for the Northern Ireland Grammar School Senior Certificate of Education; or
(4) Such other qualifications as the Council may consider the equivalent to those set out in paragraph 1 (a), (b) or (c) of this rule; or
(5) A specified pass standard in an educational test approved by the Council; or
(6) Such vocational qualifications as the Council may from time to time approve as providing a standard of education appropriate to entry into such training.

Please note the following:

(1) In accordance with Rule 16 (1) (d) the UKCC has compiled a list of acceptable alternative qualifications to those listed in 16.1 (a)–(c) for both UK and overseas applicants (see section 3.3 onwards of the handbook).

(2) The DC Educational Test series (DC1, DC2, DC3) has been approved by UKCC under Rule 16.1 (e) for entry to pre-registration programmes leading to qualification for admission to parts 1, 3, 5, 8, 12, 13, 14 and 15 of the register (see section 3.6 of the handbook).

Pre-registration first level midwifery courses

The minimum statutory requirements for entry to a pre-registration midwifery course leading to qualification on part 10 of the register are specified in Rule 30.1 (a–e) of the Nurses, Midwives and Health Visitors (Fever Nurses Amendment Rules and Training Amendment Rules) Approval Order 1989 (No. 1456).

They are not less than:

(1) A minimum of five subjects any of which may be obtained in the General Certificate of Secondary Education in England and Wales grade A, B or C, or at Ordinary level grade A, B or C in the General Certificate of Education of England and Wales, or at Grade 1 in the Certificate of Secondary Education, of which one shall be English Language and one shall be a Science subject; or

(2) A minimum of five subjects any of which may be obtained at Ordinary or Standard Grade, grade 1, 2 or 3 or at Ordinary Grade (bands A, B or C) in the Scottish Certificate of Education, of which one shall be English Language and one shall be a Science subject; or

(3) A minimum of five subjects any of which may be obtained in the General Certificate of Secondary Education in Northern Ireland, grade A, B or C, or at Ordinary level, of which one shall be English Language and one shall be a Science subject; or

(4) Such other qualifications as the Council may consider the equivalent to those set out in sub-paragraph (1), (2) or (3) of this paragraph; or

(5) A specified pass standard in an educational test approved by the Council.

The application processing system

Under normal circumstances the NMCCH will only process applications for courses which have received ENB approval. This approval is reviewed regularly to ensure the maintenance of standards. However, as an exception to the rule, there are instances where Colleges are 'awaiting' approval of certain courses, e.g. Project 2000 courses. The applicant does not apply to the NMCCH for a specific commencement date, but indicates on the application form the earliest date at which they are available for entry to a course; it is then up to the relevant College of Nursing or Midwifery to consider the applications. Providing the application meets the set criteria it will be accepted by the NMCCH and processed. If it does not, it will be withdrawn. The whole process of application takes about 5 months to complete. Once the College is in receipt of the completed application form from the NMCCH decisions are made to either interview the candidate or reject the application. It is unusual for Colleges to offer a place on a course without interviewing the candidate. If an interview is arranged it is important that the candidate takes with him or her the required documentation, e.g. usually originals are requested of Birth Certificate/Marriage Certificate, Educational Certificates, Deed Poll, etc.

Some Colleges will not interview unless the certificates are provided. The decision to interview or reject is with the College to which application has been made and not the NMCCH, which means that submitting an application form to the NMCCH does not guarantee the applicant an interview nor does attending for interview mean a place is guaranteed on the course. The applicant is not limited to applying to one College only – on the application form he or she can indicate a choice of between one and six Colleges, anywhere in the country. The NMCCH handbook refers to these choices as *first set* and *second set*. The first set choice is where the applicant *really* would like to undertake the course and these colleges receive the application form first. The second set choice will *only* receive copies if the applicant is not offered a place on any of the first set choices or if the applicant declines any offers made.

Once the completed application form is received, it is checked and – providing it is valid – the information is entered on a computer and the applicant is sent a letter acknowledging the application. Once the application is received by the NMCCH it is not possible for the candidate to alter any information except academic status/personal details.

Copies of the application form are sent to first set choices simultaneously and they have 8 weeks to consider the application, call the candidate for interview, make a decision and inform the NMCCH of their decision. (More often than not candidates are informed of the decision on the day of interview.) If offered an interview at each of the first set choices the candidate may wish to attend them all and not wish to make a decision about accepting until this is complete, or they may wish to accept an offer at any one of the interviews. If this is the case, it is the responsibility of the candidate to inform the NMCCH. If on the other hand the candidate does not wish to accept any of the offers, if made, or the Colleges do not make an offer of a place, the second set choices are sent the application forms and the process continues as in the first set choices. Whatever the decisions reached, the NMCCH does not receive any indication as to *why*. If the candidate wishes to withdraw their application at any stage, for whatever reason, he or she is at liberty to do so, but must inform the NMCCH of this decision. Offers made through the NMCCH are subject to satisfactory medical examination and clearance and also subject to no major changes in personal circumstances.

To apply through the NMCCH the prospective candidate must obtain a copy of the *The Applicant Handbook* and an application form. The handbook contains all the information required by the applicant to complete the application form. There is a nominal charge for this book which is currently £6, but a copy is usually available in the College of Nursing. It is important that the candidate completes the form accurately. The handbook is divided into sections as follows:

Section 1: guide to the NMCCH

This section gives details about the NMCCH system and how to use the book in order to complete the application form for the courses available through the NMCCH.

Section 2: careers

This section looks at the changes occurring in Nurse Education and contains information related to the Nursing/Midwifery professions and also salaries, visa requirements and opportunities.

Section 3

This section deals with the entry requirements.

Section 4

This deals with how to make an application and how it is processed.

Section 5

This section is related to health declaration forms.

Section 6

This contains the information about the Colleges offering courses.

So far in this chapter we have explored the possible avenues for progression. There will be some people who want to work within health care but not necessarily move on to the demands of further education. For those who wish to avail themselves of the opportunities, the pathways of progression will be there and with guidance and advice from the professionals involved, their educational journeys would be made as problem free as possible. The other members of this workforce who do not wish to move on, however, must not be disadvantaged in terms of provision for maintaining their skills. This is an individual choice based on

Minimum age 16½ – Apply to NMCCH (relevent fee to be paid)

↓

Receive handbook/application form

↓

Choose up to six training institutions

↙

Application form to first reference

↓

Application form returned to NMCCH

↓

Providing you are : old enough
satisfy entry requirements
and have applied for valid institution and course

↓

Application form sent to 1st three choices

↓ (first set)

Educational have eight weeks to consider your application

Accept offer	Reject offer or offer refused

Application form sent to next
three choices – second set
eight weeks to consider

↓

Unsuccessful
Enter regional clearing pool (for 1 year)
Contact local Careers Advisor

Successful – accept place

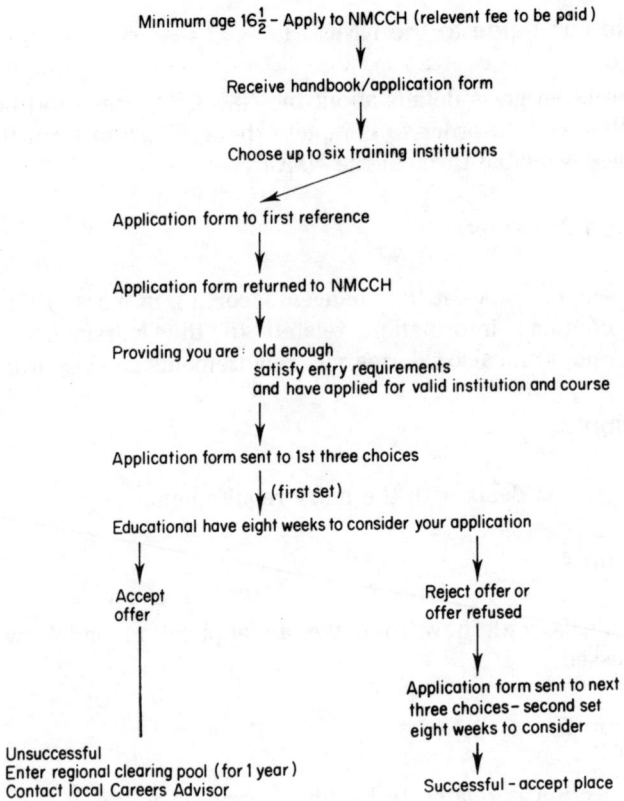

Fig. 9.3. Teaching cycle.

circumstances, and for a variety of reasons they may not wish to pursue academically orientated courses of study.

However, if the standards of care are to be maintained and improved, and also the individual's motivation maintained, a system of continuing education must be provided by the employing authority. This provision need not be a theoretical update but would probably be more appropriate in terms of improving the practical skills required in the carrying out of their role within the care team. The provision of in service training for all grades of staff from all disciplines within the caring teams is well established and the range of available courses is based on the perceived needs of the service in the local areas. The emphasis placed on this service varies but the fact that staff are provided with the facility denotes an interest on the part of their employing authority and acknowledges the valuable contribution made to health care by the staff. This interest shown helps to maintain the motivation of the staff, helping them retain an interest in their roles and giving them a sense of individual worth.

The determination of the programmes for in service training should involve the individuals concerned and their ideas should be taken into account. Some of the continuing education programmes may be done on an individual basis in the clinical area in which the Health Care Support Worker is employed. This would probably be undertaken by the qualified practitioners. If the areas of update required are common to a number of staff, then the college of nursing or the in service training department will, in consultation with the managers and qualified practitioners, design appropriate programmes. Those involved in the updating or re-skilling of supportive role staff are helping to improve the quality of care provisions.

Information sources

NMCCH. *Applicants Handbook.*
Nurse Selection Project. *Taking the DC Test: A Guide for Candidates.* School of Education, University of Leeds.

Further information

Nurse Preparation/Career Advice,

English National Board,
Careers Service,
764a Chesterfield Road,
Sheffield,
S8 OSE.

NNEB,
Argyle House,
29–31, Euston Road,
London NW1 2SD

Outside England contact addresses

Chief Nursing Officer,
Welsh Office,
Cathays Park,
Cardiff CF1 3NG

Nursing Advisor,
Scottish Health Service Centre,
Crewe Road,
Edinburgh EH4 2LF

Recruitment Officer,
National Board for Nursing, Midwifery and Health Visiting, for
  Northern Ireland,
RAC House,
79, Chichester Street,
Belfast BT1 4JE

National Boards

English National Board,
Victory House,
170, Tottenham Court Road,
London W1A OHA

National Board for Scotland,
22, Queen Street,
Edinburgh,
EH2 1JX

Northern Ireland National Board,
RAC House,
79, Chichester Street,
Belfast
BT1 4JE

Welsh National Board,
Floor 13,
Pearl Assurance House,
Greyfriars Road,
Cardiff CF1 3AG

Nurses and Midwives Central Clearing House,
English National Board,
PO Box 346,
Bristol BS99 7FB

Open and Distance Learning

Distance Learning Centre,
South Bank Polytechnic,
Room 1D35,
Southbank Technopark,
90 London Road,
London SE1 6LN

Open University,
Walton Hall,
Milton Keynes,
Buckinghamshire,
MK7 6AA

United Kingdom Central Council for Nursing, Midwifery and
    Health Visiting,
23, Portland Place,
London W1N 3AF

Continuing Nurse Education,
Barnet College,
Russel Lane,
Whetstone,
London N20 OAY

For more information contact: Open College

The Open College,
101, Wigmore Street,
London,
W1H 9AA

The Open College
3rd Floor
St. James' Buildings,
Oxford Street,
Manchester M1 6FQ

The Open College
5th Floor,
Atlantic Chambers,
45 Hope Street,
Glasgow G2 6AF

The Open College
6th Floor
Bedford House,
16–22 Bedford Street,
Belfast BT2 7FD

10

Reflections in the Pool

The issues relating to the introduction of the Health Care Support Worker are still the subject of much debate. The world of health care is constantly changing in response to the changing environment and many of the roles and functions of Health Care Workers are changing. In relation to the new worker, much has been achieved in terms of identifying what the Health Care Support Worker can and cannot do, however the defining of the actual role has yet to be done. There are many opinions voiced about the nature of the job the Health Worker should undertake. In the nursing profession this new 'helper' role is designed to assist the qualified Nurses in the delivery of care by providing much of the care which is undertaken by the present Nursing

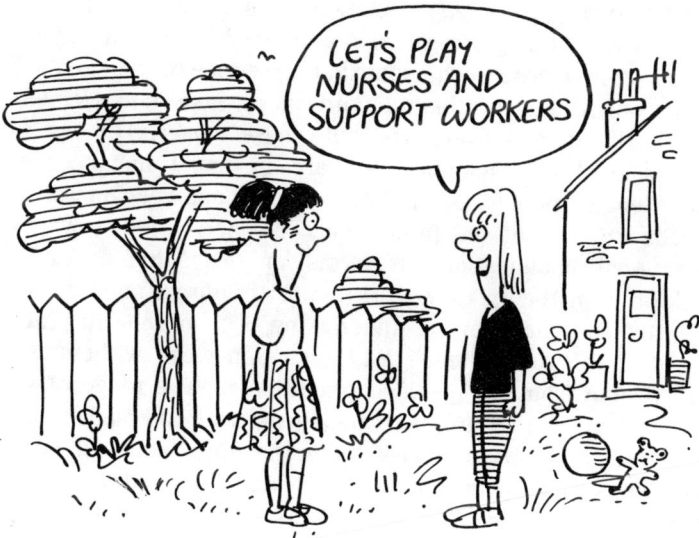

Auxiliaries. This new helper grade was identified in the United Kingdom Central Council for Nursing, Midwifery and Health Visiting (UKCC) proposal for the reform of Nurse Education *Project 2000 – A New Preparation for Practice*. The proposal was accepted by the Government on the understanding that work should be undertaken in order to widen the entry gate into Nursing and that the training and role specification of this new Health Worker grade be addressed.

Because of the changes proposed in relation to Nurse Education, fears were expressed within the NHS that the reduction in the amount of participation in the clinical areas on the part of the student nurses in training, combined with the reduction in numbers of school leavers who could be recruited, would create serious problems in terms of staffing unless a new source of recruitment could be found. The introduction of this new grade of worker has implications for the professional workforce for whom they would be providing support in relation to skill mix. This was discussed in an article in *Nursing Times* in 1987 by Dickson and Cole in which they identified that the proportion of support workers to trained staff effectively determines not only what the Support Worker can and cannot do, but also what the qualified Nurses can and cannot do.

The idea of a Support Worker is not new to the health care system, the professional practitioners having a variety of 'unqualified' workers who contribute a service to the clients. The work undertaken by this taskforce is an important element in the health care delivery systems. These workers do not hold professional qualifications, but are in many instances very experienced people. At present this is not recognized as a 'qualification', but in future may be accredited towards a vocational qualification. In terms of the Nursing Auxiliary taskforce, in theory they work under the direct supervision of the qualified Nurse in the undertaking of their role. In practice many of this 'unqualified' taskforce often work without direct supervision from the qualified practitioners. The range of work undertaken by this group of people is wide although in most areas they tend not to be involved in the more 'technical' nursing practices such as giving injections. The range of duties undertaken by those in support roles varies also and may include clerical duties, e.g. those who work in out patients' departments may combine a clerical role with a role that involves helping the qualified Nurses to assist the medical personnel. Many of this taskforce have received little or no direct training for the job in which they are employed and have learned the 'ropes' of the job by working alongside another more experienced worker. In terms of preparation for their role, this is a most unsatisfactory method and one which – the new approach to training advocated – will cease to be the norm. This situation is now being addressed and training programmes specifically designed to prepare those in support roles for their job.

In addition to this the person is offered the opportunity of gaining a nationally recognized vocational qualification, on which he or she can build, and clearly this progress in the direction of their choice in the field of health care is a step in the right direction in terms of providing a first class service. The views on the introduction of this new worker, with its potential problems, are probably as many in number as there are qualified Nurses working within the health care settings.

However, three major 'camps' have been identified. The Royal College of Nursing and many of the qualified Nurses, some of

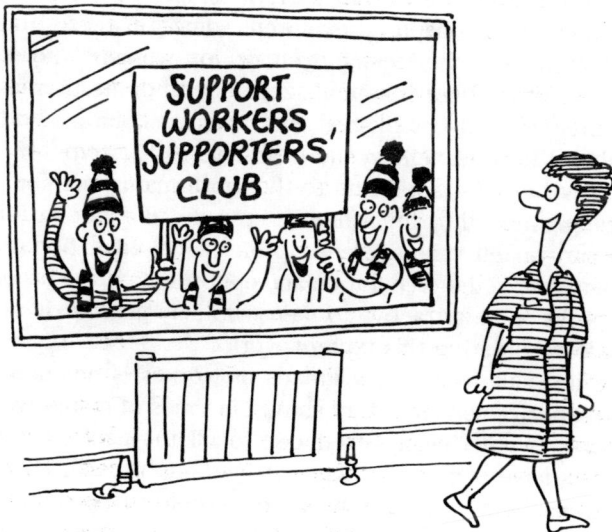

whom are noted academics, within the profession were in favour of an all-qualified nursing workforce with the trained Nurses delivering all direct nursing care. In this situation the Support Worker would undertake 'non nursing' duties such as clerical or housekeeper-type roles.

The UKCC in the Project 2000 proposals estimated that 70% of the direct care would be provided by the qualified practitioners, 28% by the unqualified Support Worker who would work under the direct supervision and monitoring of the qualified practitioner. The remaining 2% of the care would be undertaken by Student Nurses as part of the professional education courses leading to qualification as Registered Practitioners.

The remaining camp, in which the National Health Service Training Authority is included, holds the view that the highly trained practitioners, in particular the Project 2000 nurse, would need to be supported by a larger rather than smaller number of Support Workers.

Whatever role is developed for the Health Care Support Worker, and many innovative ideas are in progress with others in advanced stages of preparation, the question remains regarding recruitment. One possible route of recruitment and eventual retention is to make the proposition so attractive it tempts people to return to work. Previous chapters explored some of these routes to employment for the unemployed or for women who want to return to work following an absence due to domestic reasons. It has already been established that there will be a shortfall of suitable school leavers in the near future. This type of worker role may be more appealing to the more mature person, or the young person who, for whatever reason, did not acquire the necessary qualifications to enter professional education. Because of the nature of the preparation and opportunities, the proposition may prove to be attractive to men who may previously not have considered entering this type of work.

The introduction of new grades of worker is not new to the Nursing profession as history shows. In times of manpower crisis new grades have been introduced to fill the gaps. In the past, mistakes have been made which have been recognized only on reflection. Some of the resultant problems are still being experienced by the profession. Many professional practitioners think that the introduction of a new worker into the health care sector today may be history repeating itself. However, there is a difference in today's approach, in that it has been stated that the workers in this group will be specifically trained for the role of supporting the professional, and although they receive a qualification it is not a professional qualification. This evidently is very different from the way in which new workers were introduced in the past. Another point in favour is the possible progression of the Health Care Support Worker. There are opportunities available in terms of career structure and pathways for advancement for the individual to take advantage of.

Regarding the system of awarding National Vocational Qualifications (NVQs) there is still a considerable amount of work to be undertaken. The Joint Awarding Bodies are reviewing and amending the competencies required, and in the not too distant future we should hopefully have a system of preparing those who are to support the professional in an appropriate manner which will satisfy all concerned, including the professional practitioners.

For those who will be involved in the training of the Health Care Support Worker there is much to do in terms of preparation for the role of trainer and assessor. Training courses will be facilitated either by the Departments of Continuing Education or similar organizations in further education. It is vital that the role and training of this new worker is one in which the professional is totally involved in order to determine the extent of the support required and how this support is to be undertaken. Without involvement of the professions in this formulation of the role and function and the setting of the parameters within which the Health Support Worker will work, we are in danger of entering a revolving door which could lead to a situation, not uncommon today, where helper grades were imposed.

The opportunity is there for us, the professionals, to help shape the future. We should grasp it in both hands and not let go until we are satisfied that we have tried to get the best out of circumstances beyond our control. The actual functioning of the helper grades will be determined at local level to suit the identified needs within their health care delivery systems. The common factor will be the 'qualification' awarded by nationally recognized bodies identifying the level of competence of the individuals concerned. This indication of level of competence is important to both the practitioners and the Health Support Worker. From a prospective employer's perspective, the knowledge that an individual has demonstrated competence and been awarded a Level I or Level II NVQ is an important factor. Transferability of NVQs allows for a more mobile group of workers and affords the individual the opportunity to be selective in his or her choice of areas of health care.

Perhaps now, having dived into the pool of NVQs and gained the confidence in the water you may wish to swim further!

Some Articles of Interest

Bolger, T. (1989). Handle with Care. *Nursing Times*, May 24, **85** (21).

Dickson, N. and Cole, A. (1987). Nurse's Little Helper? *Nursing Times*, March 11th.

Fardell, J. (1989). Short Cut at Short Change? *Nursing Times*, **85** (7).

Harrison, D. (1988). Nursing Auxiliaries – an asset not to be wasted. *Senior Nurse*, **8** (3).

Johnstone, C. (1989). Who is the Support Worker? *Nursing Times*, **2** (15), 85–87.

Malby, R. (1989). Cultivate Support Workers. *Nursing Times*, **85** (26).

Malby, R. (1989). Day of the Support Worker. *Nursing Standard*, **3** (32).

Rowden, R. (1989). Helper or Hindrance? *Nursing Times*, February 22, **85** (8).

Salvage, J. (1988). In the Ghetto. *Nursing Times*, **84** (32).

Storey, L., Ruhi, H. and Behi. (1988). YTS The Question or the Answer? *Nursing Times*, August 17, **84** (33).

Index

T